OXFORD MEDICAL PUBLICATIONS

....

Children in Hospital

Children in Hospital

A Guide for Family and Carers

RICHARD LANSDOWN

Honorary Senior Lecturer,
Centre for International Child Health,
Institute of Child Health,
University of London
Formerly Consultant Psychologist
Great Ormond Street Hospital

Oxford   New York   Tokyo
OXFORD UNIVERSITY PRESS
1996

Oxford University Press, Walton Street, Oxford OX2 6DP
Oxford   New York
Athens   Auckland   Bangkok   Bombay
Calcutta   Cape Town   Dar es Salaam   Delhi
Florence   Hong Kong   Istanbul   Karachi
Kuala Lumpur   Madras   Madrid   Melbourne
Mexico City   Nairobi   Paris   Singapore
Taipei   Tokyo   Toronto
and associated companies in
Berlin   Ibadan

Oxford is a trade mark of Oxford University Press

Published in the United States
by Oxford University Press Inc., New York

A catalogue record for this book is available from the British Library

Library of Congress Cataloging in Publication Data
Lansdown, Richard.
Children in hospital : a guide for family and carers / Richard
Lansdown.
(Oxford medical publications)
Includes index.
1. Children – Hospital care.   2. Children – Preparation for medical
care.   I. Title.   II. Series.
RJ242.L36   1996   362.1'9892–dc20   95–20564
Library of Congress Cataloging in Publication Data

ISBN 0 19 2623583 (Hbk)
ISBN 0 19 2623575 (Pbk)

Typeset by EXPO Holdings, Malaysia
Printed in Great Britain by
Biddles Ltd
Guildford & King's Lynn

Foreword

by Claire Rayner

There can be few more emotive subjects than children in hospital. Just thinking about small children in clinical surroundings is enough to open the floodgates of adult tears, adult sentimentality, and often adult purse strings. When Great Ormond Street started its Wishing Well Appeal a few years ago it was over-subscribed in an incredibly short time and the money still rolls in.

This splendid book, however, opens a different set of floodgates – those of knowledge. It is one of the most fascinating texts I've read for a very long time, marrying as it does history with accounts of the most modern practice. If you're interested in the way children were cared for in illness in antiquity, there is information here. If you want to know how understanding of child illness shaped the form of care that was provided in more recent times, the facts you need are in these pages. If your interest is in the way children themselves react to illness, to pain, and to stress, go no further. If your tastes are more academic and your fascination is with the ethical issues around caring for people who, by definition, are unable on the grounds of their immaturity to make informed decisions for themselves, there is much food for thought here.

The book is described as a guide for families and carers, but it's more than that. Any person who is interested in the place children hold in our society, who is concerned with the welfare of children when they are well and not only when they are ill, will find much here to make them think. This book is child centered in the best possible sense. It is filled with a great deal of sympathy and concern for children, without being sentimental in any way. It offers a child's eye view of life and sickness without in any way being childish or simplistic, and, an added bonus in these days when the importance of the message has been allowed to dominate the manner in which it is said, it is a joy to read well written prose that is grammatical, elegant, sometimes witty, always readable. Richard Lansdown is to be congratulated on providing a text that will live on the shelves of intelligent and interested people for many years to come. It will be a brave man or woman who will try to better it.

To all those children—and their families

Acknowledgements

I would like to thank a number of people who read early drafts of chapters and made helpful comments: John Carrier, Ginny Colwell, Betty Goldsborough, Patricia Kenny, Bryan Lask, Ray Lunnon, Gillian Tindall, and Caroline Woodroffe.

The help of librarians at Action for Sick Children, the University of London Institute of Child Health, and the Charles West School of Nursing has been invaluable.

Permission to quote from the work of others is also acknowledged: Action for Sick Children for the poem by 'A.B.' (Chapter 4, p. 54) and extracts from an article by Tipping, Schwartz, and Chapman, both of which appeared in the journal *Cascade* (Chapter 18).

Nursing Standard Publications for the reproduction of the diagram on p. 111, from *Paediatric Nursing*, 6, 11–13.

Contents

Contents

1

The earliest hospitals of all

The word 'hospital' is a trap, for it has meant different things in different eras. The earliest definition given in the *Shorter Oxford English Dictionary* is 'a place of rest and entertainment'. (This chimes with the words of the mother of a patient in Great Ormond Street Hospital a few years ago: 'This place is a holiday camp—with needles.')

The first children's hospitals were, indeed, places of shelter, their inmates having been abandoned. The very first children's hospitals were probably the foundling asylums, the earliest, or at least one of the earliest, being established by Archbishop Datheus in Milan in 787, with others at Bergamo in 982 and Florence in 1161. 'Asylum' is another word which has changed in its connotations; the original meaning was an institute of shelter and support.

By the seventeenth century, the intention of the founders and the outcome of their work were frequently far apart. The places of shelter often became death houses, rapidly seeing off their charges. In 1639, for example, 75 per cent of the infants brought from the provinces to the French Hospice des Enfants Trouvés died. Just over a hundred years later the position was worse: 80 per cent of the 31 951 infants admitted between 1771 and 1777 died before the end of their first year. An enquiry instituted by Louis XIV noted eight to nine children to a bed and near total mortality. Over a similar period the Dublin Foundling Hospital had a mortality rate of 99.6 per cent (Brandon 1986).

The reasons for the death rate were not hard to find: a lack of staff, an inadequate diet, poor hygiene, and intercurrent infection took their toll, reflecting the poverty of medical knowledge of the time.

The study of paediatrics

The early years

Although the study of children's medicine could be said to have begun as early as 1500 BC, the Ebers Papyrus gives prescriptions for some diseases of childhood (including recommending an extract of poppy mixed with wasp excrement to stop an infant crying), the formal study of paediatrics took a long while to flower. The Ancient Greek physician Aretaeus mentioned children's diseases briefly in the first century AD. Around AD 30 Cornelius Celsus wrote *De re medicina* the earliest Latin medical work and was one of the first, if not the first, to make the point that 'children require to be treated entirely differently from adults' (Brandon 1986).

One has to wait until 1472 for Pietro Bagellardo of the University of Padua to publish *Libellus de egritudinibis*, the first distinct text on paediatrics. It was another hundred years before the first text appeared in English. Thomas Phaire (Phayer, Faer, Faier, or Phaer) produced *The boke of chyldren* in 1545. Phaire started with the importance of feeding; one must choose a wet nurse with care, for temperament, he asserted, is passed through the milk. He also noted the importance of contagion, in this, as in many other ways, being ahead of his time. See Table 1.1 for some details of Phaire's preoccupations.

Modern paediatrics

The foundations of modern paediatrics are said to have been laid by Rosen von Rosenstein with his 1765 *The diseases of children and their remedies*. However, the word spread slowly and as late as 1838 William Buchan observed, 'Nor have physicians themselves been sufficiently attentive to the management of children; this has been generally considered as the sole province of old women, while men of the first character in physic have refused to visit infants even when sick' (Buchan 1838). It was not just that men of the first or even second character considered medicine for children to be beneath them, it was, despite the efforts of early authors, thought to be an impossible topic to study and practice, 'since children cannot tell of their ailments and doctors are incompetent to prescribe for them' (Brandon 1986).

Traditional practices and beliefs abounded up to the nineteenth century. Disease and death were seen by many as a punishment for sin (a belief still found in some children and not a few adults). Children born at the time of the new moon were sure to prosper, while those born on a Friday were doomed to ill luck. Toothache was treated by burning a candle of mutton fat mingled with the seed of sea holly close to the tooth, holding a basin of cold water beneath, so that the worm causing the pain would fall into the water to escape the heat (King-Hall 1958).

Table 1.1   The common diseases of children, Thomas Phair

Yet for most commonly the tender age of children is chiefly vexed and greued with these diseases folowyng.

Apostume of the brayne
Swellyng of the head
Scalles of the head
Watchyng out of measure
Terryble dreams
The falling euill
The Palsey
Crampe
Styfnesse of limmes
Bloudshotten eyes
Watryng eyes
Scabbynesse and ytche
Diseases in the eares
Neasing out of measure
Bredyng of teeth
Canker in the mouth
Quinsie, or swellyng of throte
Coughe
Streytnesse of wynde
Febleness of the stomake & vomiting
Yeaxying or hicket
Colyke and rumblyng in the guttes
Fluxe of the belly
Wormes
Swelyng of the nauill
The stone
Pyssing in bedde
Brustyng
Failing of the skynne
Chafyng of the skynne
Small pockes and measels
Feuers
Swelling of the coddes
Sacer ignis or chingles
Burnyng and scaldyng
Kybbes
Consumpcion
Leaneness
Gogle eyes

The boke of chyldren, Thomas Phaire (1545).

Much is made of the horrors of poverty-stricken children's lives in the past but the upper classes were not immune. King Henry III lost five children, Edward I lost seven, and Edward III lost four.

High rates of infant mortality have been put forward to explain the lack of interest in medical treatment for children before the nineteenth century; it has been said by some that it was not only that medicine had little to offer, adults rarely became attached to their young children because their life span was expected to be short. Ariès (1973) quotes Montaigne in support of this idea: 'I have lost two or three children in their infancy, not without regret, but without great sorrow.' Stone (1977) notes 'In the 16th and early 17th century very many fathers seem to have looked on their infant children with much the same degree of affection which men today bestow on domestic pets.' Stone (1977) goes on to point out that there is no evidence, in Britain at least, of parental attendance at the funerals of very young children in the sixteenth, seventeenth, or eighteenth centuries.

It is easy to exaggerate this apparent lack of feeling. There is a reliance on selective quotations from the recorded views of the minority who could write and generalizations from this source to the whole population are questionable. The picture is made more complex by the fact that many parents, not only those from the upper classes, 'fostered out' their babies to a wet nurse for the first 2 years, perhaps to make the level of infant mortality easier to bear. They therefore had little or no contact with them; we cannot go back to ask the wet nurses how they felt when their charges died or were taken from them.

There is anecdotal evidence, also quoted in Stone (1977), that an affective bond did develop between parents and young children once the period of infancy was over. Shakespeare must have struck a chord in his audience when he wrote, in *King John*:

> Grief fills the room up of my absent child
> Lies in his bed, walks up and down with me,
> Put on his pretty looks, repeats his words,
> Remembers me of all his gracious parts,
> Stuffs out his vacant garments with his form.

It is also possible to counter the indifference argument with quotations, certainly from the eighteenth century, which suggest that the death of an infant was, indeed, frequently a matter of much emotion. When Boswell's 5-month-old son died, he wrote, 'I cried over my little son, and shed many tears' (Weis and Pottle 1970). It is hard to believe that adults of any era who have looked after an infant for even a few days will not have developed some attachment.

Hospitals and the nineteenth-century social conscience

Concern for children's health expressed in the establishment of hospitals should be seen within the context of the mid–to late nineteenth-century's general social conscience. Britain became richer and more powerful and it was a common view amongst high minded citizens that the Empire was bringing enlightenment and civilization to the heathen masses.

> From Greenland's icy mountains,
> From India's coral strand,
> Where Afric's sunny fountains
> Roll down their golden sand.
> What though the spicy breezes
> Blow soft o'er Ceylon's isle;
> From many an ancient river
> From many a palmy plain
> They call us to deliver
> Their land from error's chain.
>
> Bishop Reginald Heber (1783–1826)

In Britain the masses to be delivered were those living in poverty: ill fed, ill housed, exploited in youth, and neglected in old age, they desperately needed the legislation that came thick and fast. The 1840 Chimney Sweeps Act banned the use of children as sweeps, the 1842 Mines Act forbade the employment of women, girls, and boys under the age of 10 years underground, the 1870 Education Act brought at least the possibility of universal education, and the 1872 Life Protection Act demanded the registration and licensing of baby farms (defined as places in which children less than 1 year old were looked after for more than 1 day for payment).

The first modern hospitals for children

The forerunners

One of the last foundling hospitals, set up by the sea captain Thomas Coram in London, formed a bridge between the old idea of a refuge with the more modern concept of medical care. The main aim of the founders was still to provide some shelter to those infants who would otherwise have been murdered, exposed to perish in the streets, or trained in idleness, beggary, and theft. But the first foundling hospital's committee, set up in 1739, sought advice on the care of children from the College of Physicians. Despite the advice that might have been given, the mortality rate was 70 per cent in the first 4 years. W. Buchan, medical officer to the Ackworth branch, found 'fevers and other internal disorders ... and ... a putrid dysentery, which proved so infectious that it carried off a great many of the children' (Buchan 1838).

Another landmark came when the Dispensary for the Infant Poor was opened in Red Lion Square, London in 1769 by George Armstrong. Dispensaries, which owed their origin in the seventeenth century to the desire of physicians to hold the apothecaries at bay, were places where the poor could go for advice and medicine without having to pay for either (Cope 1964). Children were received there without letters of recommendation if need be and 35 000 were dealt with in 12 years. In Armstrong's words, 'No charitable institution was ever assembled whereby so much good has been done, or so many lives saved at so small an expense.' Unfortunately his work ended in 1781 when he ran out of money and he later died in obscurity.

In 1772 several Friends to the Charity wondered about the value of a 'House fitted up for the reception of such Infants as are very ill where they might be accommodated in the same Manner as Adults are in other Hospitals' (Maloney 1954). Armstrong would have none of this:

If you take away a sick child from its Parent or Nurse you break its Heart immediately; and if there must be a Nurse to each Child what kind of an Hospital must there be to contain any Number of them? Besides, as in this case the Wards must be crowded with grown Persons as well as Children must not the Air of the Hospital be thereby much contaminated? Would not the Mothers or Nurses be perpetually at Variance with one another if there were such a Number of them together? Would not the Children almost constantly disturb each other with their Crying ...? (Maloney 1954).

John Bunnell Davis, the founder of what became the Royal Universal Dispensary for Children, Waterloo, which was opened in 1816, had far reaching plans for the treatment of children's diseases and even more ambitious hopes, partially realized, for using his establishment for the training of doctors but he rejected children's wards as far too dangerous (Franklin 1964).

Florence Nightingale was no advocate of children's hospitals either, favouring the practice of putting young children in women's wards, as the older patients 'often became the child's best protector and nurse'. She doubted also that enough nurses could ever be found:

It is not enough to be merely conscientious and patient. There must be a real, genuine vocation and love for the work; a feeling as if your own happiness were bound up in each child's recovery. Nothing else will carry you through the perpetual wear and tear of the spirits, of the fretfulness, the unreasonableness of sick children—not that I think it is greater than that of many sick adults—but it is more wearing, because the strain is never off for a minute (Nightingale 1914).

The view prevailed. In January 1843 an enquiry in England and Wales established that only 26 children under 10 years of age 'suffering from Diseases peculiar to their age' were in hospital, at a time when London had 2363 occupied medical beds (West 1854).

Continental Europe followed a different path. In 1787 a private hospital for children was set up in Vienna and in 1792 the Parisian asylum Maison de l'Enfant Jésus became the Hôpital des Enfants Malades. Other hospitals, using the word in the modern sense, were set up in Petrograd and Berlin (1834), Hamburg (1840), Moscow, Prague, and Stuttgart (1842), Turin (1843), Stockholm (1845), Copenhagen (1946), and Constantinople (1847). (See Garrison (1965) for details.)

Great Ormond Street

Britain could not hold out for long. Founded in 1722, Guy's Hospital had from the beginning admitted children to the women's wards, but from 1831 they had 15 cribs for children in a wooden building over some stables. Unfortunately these were not replaced when the building was pulled down in 1850. However, this kind of provision was far from a separate hospital for children. In 1850 the matter was addressed, when a meeting of nine 'gentlemen desirous of promoting a hospital for sick children' was held in Lower Grosvenor Street. This meeting was driven by the vision of Dr Charles West, physician to the Royal Universal Dispensary for Children. West had travelled in France and Germany and had written to a great many continental hospitals. Having failed to convert the Waterloo Road Dispensary into an in-patient institution he and his committee colleagues finally lighted upon 49 Great Ormond Street, a house which was rented, for £200 per annum for 21 years, on 29 April 1851. The original name given to this new institution was The London Hospital for Sick Children but by November it was noted that confusion was arising with The London Hospital and the 'London' was dropped. With 10 beds, the first patients were admitted on St Valentine's Day, 14 February 1852, the doors being opened 'quietly, without ceremony' by the porter. It is possible that St Valentine's day was not the opening day (Kosky 1992; J. Kosky, personal communication) but that is the popular belief. Great Ormond Street was, then, the first children's hospital with beds to be opened in Britain. (See Appendix 1 for a list of others.)

The aims of the hospital were set out by the provisional committee as follows (Higgins 1952).

1. To provide for the reception and maintenance and medical treatment of the children of the poor during sickness and to furnish them with advice, i.e. the mothers of those who cannot be admitted into the Hospital.

2. To promote the advancement of medical science generally with reference to the diseases of children, and in particular to provide for the more efficient instruction of students in this department of medical knowledge.

3. To disseminate among all classes of the community, but chiefly among the poor, a better acquaintance with the management of infants and children during illness by employing it as a school for the education and training of women in the special duties of children's nursing.

From the outset there were some restrictions on who could be admitted. The regulations first defined those who were accepted.

1. Children of both sexes between the ages of 2 and 12 years suffering from acute or chronic, external or internal, general or local illness.

2. Infants and children under 2 years of age are not generally eligible for admission as in-patients, it being undesirable on account of their tender age to separate them from their mothers. Such young children, however, are eligible as out-patients and, under special circumstances (to be recorded in a book kept for the purpose which shall be laid before the next meeting of the management committee), may be received into the hospital with or without their mothers.

3. Children suffering from accidents or external injuries or their immediate effects are not in general eligible as in-patients, the hospital being intended for children suffering from diseases peculiar to or modified in some important respect by their early age.

Other hospitals

The Liverpool Institution for the Diseases of Children, opened in March 1851, admitted in-patients in 1856, by which time the name had been changed to the Liverpool Infirmary for Children. On 5 February 1860, once again 'without any special ceremony' the first out-patients were admitted to the Royal Hospital for Sick Children in Edinburgh and in June 1873, also 'without ceremony' the first out-patients were admitted to a voluntary hospital in Belfast, in-patients coming a couple of months later. Quite why those recording the early days of these places were so taken with the absence of ceremony is not clear (Calwell 1973).

Other hospitals were opened in Norwich, Glasgow, Manchester, Birmingham, Gloucester, Nottingham, and Brighton.

In the United States the first children's hospital was established in Philadelphia in 1856, although there continued to be a powerful argument against such institutions; Walker Gill Wylie, winner of the Harvard Boylston Prize in 1876 for the study of hospitals, believed the bonds of the family to be threatened when sick members were removed from their houses.

The patients

The refusal by Great Ormond Street generally to admit children under the age of 2 years was followed by others, for example in Belfast, where it was not until 1896 that infants were admitted. St Mary's Hospital, Manchester, however, noted in 1857 that '... where the children are of a tender age and require maternal care, the mothers have been and will in future be admitted to take charge of and suckle such infants' (Young 1964).

The emphasis on the children of the poor noted in the Great Ormond Street aims was repeated elsewhere. The circular setting out the rationale for building a children's hospital in Belfast included the statement, 'The sick child of poor families is inevitably neglected at home. It does not know what ails it, and makes no complaint, and nobody, not even the overworked mother, has leisure to attend to it ... The child huddles into a corner, where it pines and wastes to death, or is laid hold of for life by some incurable and painful disease.'

There was, indeed, an attempt to ensure that only the poor benefited in Belfast. 'All deserving patients will be prescribed for, and get medicines gratuitously, and those bringing letters from Clergymen of any and every denomination will be promptly and especially attended to, inasmuch as their recommendation will be some guarantee of their fitness for the benefit of the charity.' It was understood that those who could afford to pay were not fit for this benefit. In Edinburgh treatment was free but parents were expected to bring their own bottles for medicine. At least one London hospital, the North Eastern (later to become the Queen Elizabeth Hospital for Children) charged 2d per patient as a matter of principle, to put off those who came for the excitement of a bottle of medicine (Kosky 1992).

A commentator in the early days of Sheffield's hospital remarked on the 'lamentable and fatal ignorance' of mothers and the great benefits of proper food and regular feeding. Clean surroundings, good nursing, and an adequate diet probably did more good than the pharmacopoeia of the time: antipyretics, antispasmodics, diuretics, expectorants, purgatives, sedatives, and tonics, this list having been taken from John McCaw's *Aids to the diseases of children* published in 1893 (Calwell 1973).

The apparent exclusion of the well to do can, therefore, partly be explained: if all one could really offer of value was a clean bed, fresh air, and good food, then what was there to attract a family which already had all three?

The food offered in hospitals may, incidentally, have been better than that available at home. Scurvy and rickets were common since fresh fruit and vegetables were thought indigestible by children, but even in 1867 the children of Great Ormond Street had green vegetables just once a week and then only if they were not too expensive. In 1877 the Sheffield Children's Hospital diet table had some vegetables but no fruit.

Common diseases of the time

The commonest diseases of patients admitted to Belfast Hospital in the first 7 months of its existence were bronchitis, pyrexia, tuberculosis, enlargement of glands, and hip and spinal diseases. Tuberculosis headed the list of causes of morbidity, syphilis was diagnosed in 28 of the first 1617 children, and only 10 cases of rickets were recorded.

There was more than a little reluctance to admit children with infectious diseases; Southampton's Shirley Hospital expressly forbade them. Such diseases formed the biggest part of Edinburgh's load with typhoid being a major factor: 11 cases in 1862 rising to 48 (with three deaths) in 1878.

Daily life in the early hospitals

The 1850s Great Ormond Street was not without its problems. There was no mains water, the cisterns were insufficient, and the kitchen boilers too weak to provide enough hot water, not surprisingly since they were designed for a private home. The drainage of the time left much to be desired and there were frequent notes by visiting governors complaining of 'an unpleasant smell'.

Charles West was described as 'not a happy colleague'. William Jenner, the other medical officer at Great Ormond Street, stares from his portrait as though rehearsing the role of Count Dracula. To be fair to him, although he frightened many adults, 'When he was with children all the goodness in him seemed to well out from him to them' (Higgins 1952). What is more, if a nurse was unable to make children happy she could be dismissed from Great Ormond Street. Further testimony of sensitivity was suggested in the care taken over the arrangements for 'the dead house'.

Treatment

It is less easy to trace with certainty what methods of treatment were used. The managers of the Massachusetts General Hospital admitted that in the 1870s it was largely a shelter providing no medical services not available in the average home (Abel Smith 1964). In the last analysis it was 'merely a nursery for sick children'. But it would be unwise to minimize the role of the carefully run shelter.

Surgery was not high in the priorities of many of these early hospitals. Great Ormond Street's Dr West and others thought, when that institution's staff was being planned, that there were no surgical problems in childhood demanding special skills or study and concluded that no surgeon should be appointed to the staff (Higgins 1952).

Staffing

The first medical staff at Great Ormond Street did in fact include a surgeon, along with two physicians, all appointed in January 1852. Later in 1852 the first resident, Mr Lynch, known as the house surgeon was appointed. He was not paid any salary but was allowed to sleep in the board room. (The porter slept in the hall.) The first dispenser was, however, paid.

The importance of nurses can be judged by the fact that the first Great Ormond Street matron, Mrs Willey, was appointed before any of the medical staff. Her opposite number in Edinburgh, a Mrs Hay, was described by an 1864 observer as, 'truly ... like the universal mother of this large and helpless family' (Calwell 1973).

The person specification for a nurse at Great Ormond Street was formidable.

As the duty of attending on sick children calls not only for the ordinary amount of patience, gentleness and kindness necessary in the case of all sick persons, but also for a freedom from prejudice and a quickness of observation seldom found among the entirely uneducated, no woman is to be admitted as a nurse who cannot read writing as well as printing, and who cannot repeat the Lord's Prayer and the Ten Commandments, and who is not acquainted with the principles of the Christian Religion, and that no one be admitted to the office of sister who is not able, in addition to the above qualifications, to write a legible hand. Further that it be the duty of every nurse not only to watch the children with care and to tend them with kindness but also to try by all means to keep them cheerful and contented (Higgins 1952).

One change in the nursing establishment was soon forced upon the Great Ormond Street administration. At first the nurse in charge of the ward at night worked alone and, as she was expected to sleep on the ward, it was not uncommon for her to fall asleep on duty. She was soon supplied with help.

Nurses had to know their place. In a book first published anonymously in 1854 entitled *How to nurse sick children* Charles West wrote:

First, however, I must remind you that a nurse is not the doctor; that she never can be; that if she forgets her proper place, and tries to interfere with his duties, or to set herself above his directions, instead of being a blessing she will be a curse, instead of promoting the sick child's recovery she will very often hasten its death (West 1854).

Early results

There were evident rewards for all this activity. Of the 25 cases first admitted to the Shirley Children's Hospital, Southampton in 1864, all 11 medical cases went home cured. Two of the surgical patients were only improved and three were still in hospital 11 months later. Speaking in 1867, Lord Dufferin saw four distinct benefits of a children's hospital.

1. The absolute good done to children

2. The admirable opportunity ... to those young women who wish to fit themselves for service in the nurseries of the upper classes.

3. Facilities for the medical profession for studying infantile disorders.

4. Moral training and religious education.

Within a year of the Royal Belfast Hospital for Sick Children having been opened in 1873 a report was made noting that

... many cases have been brought to them, in which, by timely medical treatment, perfect cures have been affected of diseases which, had they been left neglected, must have resulted in deformity or early death ... Many cases of acute disease have been brought to the hospital, in which a few days' treatment and care have been sufficient to effect cures which, under other circumstances, would probably never have been accomplished, and it has often been a source of much pain to your medical officers to be obliged to send away such cases in consequence of the limited number of beds (Calwell 1973).

Emotional factors: the nineteenth-century view of separation

The misgivings that had been felt about separating children from their parents were pacified. A Mrs Craik, visiting Edinburgh, noted in 1864,

The difficulty, which some energetic adversaries of children's hospitals have upheld so strongly—that of removing a child from home and parents—has not, in the practical working of this hospital ... been found to be a difficulty at all. For, among the classes for which it was chiefly intended, home is no home, and parents, instead of being a child's best guardian in health or sickness, are often, through ignorance and neglect, its very worst (Calwell 1973).

A more positive recommendation for the benefits of hospital came in the *Strand Magazine* of 1891:

We want now to move Johnny to a place where are none but children; a place set up on purpose for sick children; where the good doctors and nurses pass their lives with children, talk to none but children, touch none but children, comfort and cure none but children.

Who does not remember that chapter in *Our mutual friend*. Johnny is dead but the hospital in Great Ormond Street still exists—in a finer form than Dickens knew it—and still receives sick children to be comforted and cured by its gentle nurses and good doctors. From the first ward we seek to enter we are admonished by our senses to turn back. We have barely looked in when the faint, sweet odour of chloroform hanging in the air, the hiss of the antiseptic spray machine, and the screens placed round a cot informs us that one of the surgeons is conducting an operation. The ward is all hushed in silence, for the children are quick to learn that when the big, kind-eyed doctor is putting a little comrade to sleep in order to do some clever thing to him to make him well, all must be quiet as mice. There is no more touching evidence of the trust and faith of childhood than the readiness with which these children surrender themselves without a pang of fear into the careful hands of the doctor. Sometimes, when an examination or operation is over, there is a flash of resentment, as in the case of the poor boy who, after having submitted patiently to have his lungs examined, exclaimed to the doctor, 'I'll tell my mother you've been a-squeezing of me!'

We ... enter the ward called after Queen Victoria ... On the left, not far from the door, we come upon a pretty and piteous sight ... In a cot lies 'Daisy'. Her eyes open, but she does not move when we look at her; she only continues to cuddle to her bosom her brush and comb, from which the nurse tells us, she resolutely refuses to be parted ... We look round the ward and note how architectural art and sanitary and medical skill have done their utmost to make this as perfect a place as can be contrived for the recovery of health ... And what does not medical and nursing skill do for them? And tender human kindness, which is as nourishing to the ailing little ones as mother's milk ... And what a delight it must be to have constantly on your bed wonderful picture books, and on the tray that slides along the top rails of your cot the whole animal creation trooping out of Noah's Ark, armies of tin soldiers and the wonderful woolly dogs with amazing barks concealed in their bowels, or—if you happen to be a girl—dolls, dressed and undressed, of all sorts and sizes ... Until he had been in a children's hospital, no one would guess how thoughtful and good-tempered and contented a sick child can be amid his strange surroundings ... It is a constant tale of children innocently and cheerfully bearing the punishment of the neglect, the mistakes, or the sins of their parents or of society ... Our guide points out to us a little boy sitting up at the head of the couch ... He is one of the very few children who are afraid of a doctor, and he sees men there so seldom that every man appears to him a doctor ... But we cannot leave them without a final word to our readers ... let us show our pity and our admiration in such practical ways as are open to us.

The story of Daisy and others like her, is taken up in the next chapter.

References

Abel Smith, B. (1964). *The hospitals 1800–1948.* Heinemann, London.

Ariès, P. (1973). *Centuries of childhood.* Penguin Books, Harmondsworth.

Brandon, S. (1986). *Children in hospital.* National Association for the Welfare of Children in Hospital, London.

Buchan, W. (1838). *Domestic medicine.* John McGowan, London.

Calwell, H.G. (1973). *The life and times of a voluntary hospital.* Brough, Cox & Dunn, Belfast.

Cope, Z. (1964). The history of the dispensary movement. In *The evolution of hospitals in Britain,* (ed. F.N.L. Poynter). Pitman Medical Publishing, London.

Franklin, A.W. (1964). Children's hospitals. In *The evolution of hospitals in Britain,* (ed. F.N.L. Poynter). Pitman Medical Publishing, London.

Garrison, G.F. (1965). *History of paediatrics.* Dawsons of Pall Mall, London.

Garrison, W.T. and McQuiston, S. (1989). *Chronic illness during childhood and adolescence.* Sage Publications, London.

Higgins, T.W. (1952). *Great Ormond Street.* Odhams Press, London.

King-Hall, M. (1958). *The story of the nursery.* Routledge & Kegan Paul, London.

Kosky, J. (ed.) (1992). *Queen Elizabeth Hospital for Children.* The Hospitals for Sick Children, London.

Kosky, J. and Lunnon, R.J. (1991). *Great Ormond Street and the story of medicine.* Hospital for Sick Children in association with Granta Editions, London.

Maloney, W.J. (1954). *George and John Armstrong of Castledon.* E. & S. Livingstone, Edinburgh.

Nightingale, F. (1914). *Notes on nursing.* Harrison & Son, London.

Stone, L. (1973). *The family, sex and marriage.* Weidenfeld and Nicolson, London.

Weis, C.McC. and Pottle, F.A. (ed.) (1970). *Boswell in extremes, 1776–1778.* Quoted in Stone, L. (1973). *The family, sex and marriage.* Weidenfeld and Nicolson, London.

West, C. (1854). *How to nurse sick children.* Longman, Brown, Green and Longmans, London. (First published anonymously.)

Wille, J.A. (1985). From mini adult to child. Unpublished MSc thesis. Polytechnic of the South Bank, London.

Young, J.H. (1964). *St Mary's Hospital Manchester 1790–1963.* E. & S. Livingstone, Edinburgh.

2

From the battle of the visitors to the present day

Any number of influences combined to shape the development of children's hospitals in the first half of the twentieth century; any number of factors came together to bring massive change in the second half.

Medicine itself changed. An increased understanding of antiseptic and aseptic techniques gave confidence to those who thought that Science, with a capital S, was everything. Doctors became specialized, looking to the laboratory as the source of progress, and there was an emphasis on reducing complex phenomena to simple parts, studying less and less in more and more detail. The result was a more aggressive, interventionist attitude and a loss of the perception of the patient as a person (Brandon 1986). Doctors rose in social status as their craft became more esoteric and in some quarters their word became law.

The combination of this 'doctor (and by extension, nurse) knows best' attitude, plus concern about cross-infection, steadily eroded the caretaking role of mothers in hospitals and led to parents being more or less totally excluded not only from the care of their children but also from any contact at all.

The condoning of the separation of child from family was pushed along by the increase in the numbers of middle class children being admitted. Now that well-to-do parents thought that hospitals could cure, they were eager, not surprisingly, to use them. These parents shared a value system with the establishment of the time, a system which was alien to the poorer families, inconceivable to many foreigners, and perplexing to their later twentieth-century counterparts. It regarded children as beings only rarely to be seen or heard by their parents and other elders. The American psychologist J.B. Watson advised, in a book on the care of infants and children, 'Never hug and kiss them, never let them sit on your lap. If you must, kiss them once on the forehead when they say goodnight.' Later in the same book he advocated a system where each home is supplied with well-trained staff so that the babies could be fed and bathed each week by a different nurse (Watson 1928).

Among the middle to upper classes (and doctors were, of course, in this category) a tidal wave of child apartheid swept over Britain in the late nineteenth century; children were valued but kept separate, segregated first in the nursery and then looked after by governesses if they were girls and in boarding schools if they were boys. This attitude fitted neatly with the hierarchical class system that pervaded every aspect of life at this time: people knew their places and children had to imbibe the rules.

Children in hospital followed the same pattern: they needed care but were better off without contact with their parents. With no one but children to attend to, nurses could ensure that beds were neat (mitred corners to the sheets, pillow cases all facing in the same direction) and that children were docile, especially when the doctor came round. There was evidence to support this view: when parents visited and then left, children were upset—so it was better that they did not visit. When left alone children were sometimes distressed at first but they soon settled down and remained remarkably quiet for the rest of the admission. As late as 1950 a state registered nurse, speaking at a conference held by the National Federation of Women's Institutes, stated that she had never known a case of hardship caused by separation.

There were exceptions to this admittedly rather extremely presented picture. James Nicholl, a Glasgow surgeon, spoke at the British Medical Association's Annual Meeting in 1909 and argued that whenever possible children under 2 years should be treated only as outpatients. Small children 'do best in their mother's arms, and rest there more quietly on the whole than anywhere else'. He went on

For seven years I have had a small house, near the Glasgow Children's Hospital, for the accommodation of young infants and their mothers. The mothers are catered for, and themselves nurse their infants. My experience of the cases so treated has been such as to make me confident in the opinion that no children's hospital can be considered complete which has not, in the hospital or hard by, accommodation for a certain number of nursing mothers whose infants require operation.

In the 1920s, James Spence, working in the Babies Nursery in Newcastle, admitted more and more babies as in-patients; in 1925 he adapted a room to allow a mother to re-establish breast-feeding. As Brandon (1986) concluded:

Spence saw parenthood as an opportunity for personal growth and to some degree idealised the mother. His experience of mothers coping in the most adverse circumstances convinced him of the strength and effectiveness of maternal feelings in caring for and protecting her child.

The open visiting campaign

In 1949 the Central Health Services Council found that only 130 out of 1300 hospitals taking children allowed daily visiting, with 150 forbidding all visits.

In 1967 the cause of a child's death in a British hospital was given as a broken heart, his condition being diagnosed by a psychiatrist as 'severe separation anxiety'.

The years following the Second World War saw the beginning of a great many changes in Britain. Although the class system has remained intact there has been a breaking down of the more rigid hierarchies and an increasing interest in the rights of individuals. There has also been a shift from the reductionist approach in medicine towards one in which all aspects of the patient, not only the presenting symptoms, are to be addressed.

These years saw also the beginning of what became an unstoppable campaign to open up hospitals so that contact between children and their families could be maintained. Academic studies gave support to individuals and groups who between them gradually wore down opponents; it was a long struggle.

Studies on separation

A possibly apocryphal story has it that Frederik II, Holy Roman Emperor (1194–1250) was one of the first to study the effects of separating a baby from a mother. To discover what language children would speak if no-one spoke to them he had some babies cared for by foster mothers and nurses who suckled their charges but said nothing. The experiment was not a success for all the babies died, unable to live 'without petting and joyful faces and loving words' (Doxiadis 1970).

The first post-war studies were largely observational. One came from the psychoanalyst René Spitz, whose 1945 paper was a seminal work. Significantly in the light of what was subsequently done in Britain, Spitz (1945) pioneered direct observation and photography as a means of studying mother–child interactions and the film '*Grief, A Peril in Infancy*' was an early illustration of the dangers besetting separation. A paper by Prugh *et al.* (1953) demonstrated that children between 2 and 4 years of age, admitted to medical wards in America showed more immediate reactions to the experience than older children. High levels of anxiety, anger, fear, protests at separation from parents, panic, and prolonged periods of crying were described. When the children were followed up over a 6 month period the children from a 'humanized' ward showed no significant disturbance, in contrast to 15 per cent of those from a control group in an orthodox ward.

Schaffer and Callender (1959) added to the debate with their observation that a period of increased vulnerability to the effects of hospitalization could be observed in children over 6 months of age. This has led some commentators to argue that hospitalization under the age of 6 months is of little psychological consequence. Work with children with asthma does not support this view: Mrazek *et al.* (1982) found that these children's early hospital experience was not isolated or circumscribed; rather it was associated with a more subdued and passive style of interaction when children were evaluated during their preschool years compared with children with later onset asthma.

John Bowlby and attachment theory

It is almost impossible to exaggerate the importance of the next contributor to the debate. John Bowlby was a British psychiatrist whose legacy to our understanding of children was immense. One of the few writers to have contributed to theory as well as practice, his work on attachment has often been misinterpreted but has stood the test of time. It started in 1950 when he was appointed by the World Health Organization (WHO) to study the needs of children who were homeless in their native countries. In 1951 his WHO monograph *Maternal care and mental health* was published, followed by a paperback written for the general public entitled, *Child care and the growth of love* (1952). This work dealt with mother–child separation in general and carried the message that the foundation of a mentally healthy adulthood is the creation and maintenance of a warm, continuous, and mutually satisfying attachment between the infant/young child and the mother. If the attachment is not achieved or if separation brings a break, then damage ensues. Bowlby then gave theory to support the observational work of Spitz (1945) and Prugh *et al.* (1953).

Along with Bowlby, another major figure at the Tavistock Centre in London was James Robertson, a social worker appointed in 1948 to study the reactions of young children separated from their mothers. Working with his wife, Joyce, he observed children in acute and long-stay wards and, as well as writing up his results, he made the classic film *A Two Year Old Goes to Hospital* (1952). It was Robertson who identified the three stages of separation: protest, despair, and detachment (Robertson and Robertson 1989).

The initial response to this film, when shown at the Royal Society of Medicine, was hostile: this was an atypical child, with atypical parents. The paediatricians and nurses who had been invited were confident that *their* wards were happy places, for no parent complained. There was, fortunately, one exception. Ivy Morris, ward sister at Amersham General Hospital, pointed out to Dermod McCarthy, the paediatrician there, that he was wrong to dismiss the Robertsons' views. McCarthy, who was already liberal by the standards of the 1950s, took the sister's words to heart and became a champion of open visiting. It was in his hospital that Robertson made a subsequent film, *Going to Hospital with Mother.*

The movement strengthens

Notice of the psychological damage done to children was not restricted to the scientific community. At the 1950 meeting of the National Federation of Women's Institutes already referred to, children were described as returning home, 'strange, silent beings, feeling that their mothers did not love them'. At that meeting, a motion was passed deploring the fact that in some hospitals mothers were not permitted to visit their children, asking the hospital committees to allow visiting in agreement with doctors and nurses.

In the same year, an article by Sands (1950), from the Royal National Orthopaedic Hospital, Stanmore, noted that much of the objection to parental visiting came because of fears of infection. That hospital had allowed visiting three times a week for the past 18 months and found no increase in infection 'but the happiness of the children has markedly changed' (Sands 1950).

By 1951 the number of paediatric units allowing either no visiting or visiting less than once a week was 42 per cent (Institute of Child Health and Society of Medical Officers of Health and Population 1954).

Nineteen fifty-six saw the setting up, by the Central Health Services Council of the Ministry of Health, of the committee to make recommendations on the welfare of children in hospital and in February 1959 the Platt Report was accepted by the ministry. Dealing with children up to the age of 16 years, it recommended that visiting should be unrestricted and that provision should be made for mothers of children under 5 years to accompany them into hospital to help in their care and to prevent the distress of separation. Copies were sent to all hospitals admitting children. The recommendations were clear government policy but no directives accompanied the report and the struggle continued.

In 1961 a father wrote to a newspaper, 'Visiting was only an hour a day. In a few days our six month old baby had lost his identity, his eyes were 'dead' and his general appearance was of a whipped dog. It was heart breaking that after only a few days he seemed not to recognise his mother, yet was distressed at parting' (The *Guardian* 29 January 1961).

These words came as reinforcement to the four mothers who had, a year earlier, founded the group known as Mother Care for Children in Hospital. Their first annual meeting was held on 23 May 1963 with papers from paediatricians and a nurse and in May 1965 the group changed their name to the National Association for the Welfare of Children in Hospital. In 1991 the name was again changed, to Action for Sick Children.

The assertions were not all one way. In a letter to The *Guardian*, 26 July 1961, a state registered nurse and mother of four children wrote

Tell your child beforehand that he is going to stay in hospital for a few days to be made better and then calmly and with full confidence hand him over to the nursing staff. I have never seen a nurse treat a sick child with anything but the greatest care and kindness. I am still amazed at the wonderful courage and adaptability of small children. They live in the present, and if the child is going to be in hospital for a few days it is often kinder if the parents keep away.

Mothers of sick children, she went on, are 'always anxious and nervous and cannot fail to transmit some of these emotions to her child'.

In 1964 the Ministry of Health claimed that unrestricted visiting had risen to 75 per cent, a figure taken with a pinch of salt by Mother Care for Children in Hospital whose own survey put the total at something closer to 25 per cent. One explanation for the discrepancy in findings is in the differences in definition of the word 'unrestricted'. A paediatrician, quoted in The *Guardian* (23 September 1964), noted that 'Although visiting in this hospital is unrestricted we do not permit it in the mornings.'

Government action was possibly slower than it might have been due to the vociferous antagonism to unrestricted visiting that came from some very senior professionals in the field. Spence, quoted above in supporting the idea of mothers coming into hospital to breast-feed, was, however, by no means a supporter of unrestricted visiting, nor did he always show concern for the well-being of the child. In a notorious outburst at the 1951 Annual Conference of the British Paediatric Association, in Windermere, he dismissed James Robertson's notion of children being emotionally upset thus: 'What is wrong with emotional upset? This year we are celebrating the centenary of the birth of Wordsworth, the great Lakeland poet. He suffered from emotional upset, yet look at the wonderful poems he produced.' In later writing Robertson noted that this attack was probably aimed indirectly at psychiatry rather than the ideas under discussion for in his last few months Spence encouraged his students to follow Robertson's techniques of studying children.

To Sir Alan Moncrieff, physician at Great Ormond Street, first dean of the Institute of Child Health, Bowlby and Robertson were prejudiced, the hypothesis that separation brings psychological harm was unfounded, and the idea of increasing parental visiting was unwise. In a paper published in 1962 he argued that there was no evidence for the long-term effects of separation and that one should look to other variables such as whether the child came from a happy home and whether preparation had been adequate. He joined with Spence in thinking that since adversity strengthens character, separation may even be helpful: 'a part of life and even a process in development which is essential and important'. To Moncrieff, the key lay in the parents themselves, especially in the anxiety and guilt feelings of the mother.

In Moncrieff's defence it must be said that he did not always behave as the above quotations would make one imagine: in a letter to the *Lancet*, 29 January 1966, Otto Wolff, also from Great Ormond Street, pointed out that Moncrieff and his ward sister had actually encouraged unrestricted visiting for a long time.

Another landmark came with the publication of a follow-up study by James Douglas (1975) of adolescents who had been in hospital as children. (It would have been interesting to have heard Moncrieff's comments on that publication.) The database was a cohort of 3000 young people who had been examined, physically and psychologically, every 2 years since they were born in March 1946. They were in hospital at a time when visiting was severely restricted. Ten per cent of the 958 children admitted under the age of 5 years had been on adult wards, 47 per cent were allowed no visiting at all, and only three mothers stayed in with their children. Those children admitted only once before the age of 5 years for less than 1 week did seem to have been adversely affected. Admissions of more than 1 week's duration or repeated admissions before the age of 5 years (in particular between 6 months and 4 years) were associated with an increased risk of behaviour disturbance and poor reading. The children who had experienced these early admissions were not only more troublesome in school, they were more likely to be delinquent and to have unstable job patterns. Children who were over 6 years old on their first admission appeared not to have been unduly affected.

Douglas's (1975) results could not be explained by social class factors, nor by any persisting disability which might be seen to have interfered with children's education. Only children were more vulnerable than those with siblings, as were those whose mothers had just returned to work. Much less at risk were those who had been in hospital for an operation rather than for a medical reason. One explanation for this is that young children can more easily understand the reasons for being in hospital when they have to have surgical treatment than when they have a medical problem; when they could impose a meaning on their experience it made it easier to offset the pain of having been deserted by their parents.

A particularly significant finding from this study was that children showing later disturbance did not necessarily show symptoms while they were on the wards.

Although the associations were consistent with predictions that could have been made from attachment theory, Douglas (1975) pointed out that they were not necessarily causal, only 'highly suggestive ... There is the possibility that children admitted to hospital were also selected on the basis of family or environmental factors which we did not record.' Since experimental manipulation of separation in humans is unethical one has to look to animal work to provide support for the notion that separation is causally related to adverse outcome. Hinde and Davies (1972) had recently published reports of infant monkeys who had been separated from their mothers experimentally.

A relatively brief separation was followed by changes in behaviour that could be detected even two years after the reunion ... The severity was related to both type and length of separation ... Lastly, the nature and degree of the disturbance of the infant after separation was related to the adequacy of his relations to his mother before the event.

This final observation was in accord with the findings of Prugh *et al.* (1953) and colleagues already mentioned.

Douglas's (1975) paper caused a considerable stir. Quinton and Rutter (1976) replicated the study and found, also, that while a single admission, even under the age of 5 years, did not increase the risk of later psychiatric disorder, multiple admissions were associated with subsequent emotional and conduct disorders. They looked also at some of the family factors that Douglas (1975) had touched on and found that the effects were, indeed, greater among children who were vulnerable for other reasons, for example, if they were living in a broken home, if their mother had a psychiatric disturbance, or if the family were living in severely overcrowded circumstances. Even in the absence of such factors, however, the effects stood up when children who had been in hospital were compared with those who had not, although children from disadvantaged homes were more likely to have had multiple admissions (Quinton and Rutter 1976).

The blanket acceptance by psychologists of the ideas on the long-term effects quoted above has not been universal. The British psychologists Clarke and Clarke (1976) argued that associations between early separation and later disturbance can be explained in this as in any other context as illustrations not of the separation causing the difficulties, rather they are 'a sensitive index of other experiences which might lead to these difficulties'.

Further support for the long-term effects of hospitalization came, however, from Haslum (1988). She found associations between the length of time children spent in hospital before the age of 5 years and performance on vocabulary tests at 5 and 10 years and between the number of admissions and anxious behaviour at 5 years. Children whose first admission occurred between 2 and 5 years were particularly vulnerable. There was also a relationship between the length of the pre-school admission and reading and mathematics at 10 years. In an even longer term study, Pilowsky *et al.* (1982) found a higher frequency of depression and chronic illness in adults with histories of early hospitalization.

Developments elsewhere

The Association for the Care of Children's Health was founded in the United States in 1965 and during the last 30 years many similar organizations have grown up, each adding weight to the others. Examples are the Association for the Welfare of Children in Wales, the Scottish

National Association for the Welfare of Children in Hospital, the National Association for Children and Hospitals in Holland, the Nordic Association for the Care of Sick Children, the Action Committee for Children in Hospital in Germany, the Australian Association for the Welfare of Children in Hospital, and L'Association pour l'Amelioration des Conditions d'Hospitalisation des Enfants in France.

The years since 1975

The years since 1975 have seen a steady increase in open visiting in Britain and elsewhere. The Court Report (Department of Health and Social Security Committee on Child Health Services 1976) supported 'the belief of NAWCH (The National Association for the Welfare of Children in Hospital) in the value of unrestricted visiting by parents, relatives, older brothers and sisters, and school friends and the need to have sufficient rooms able to accommodate a parent or other relative with simple domestic facilities nearby'. A survey of hospitals in Wales carried out in 1981 looked at the practices of 35 hospitals admitting children, of which 28 replied. Twenty-six of them allowed unrestricted visiting for parents and 30 had accommodation of some sort for mothers to stay overnight. In 1985 a survey of Scottish wards nursing acute patients found that half had unrestricted parental visiting, with three-quarters allowing brothers and sisters as well. The majority could accommodate parents overnight.

A disturbing finding of both the above surveys was the number of hospitals admitting children to adult/mixed wards: 11 in Wales and more than half in Scotland. The most recent figures for England are from a 1987 publication and show that 26 per cent of children were still admitted to adult/mixed wards (Brittish Paediatric Association *et al.* 1987).

The picture in other countries is variable. An enquiry carried out in Massachusetts showed a rise in 24 hour visiting from 16 per cent in 1973 to 100 per cent in 1982. However a 1988 report from the American Association for the Care of Children's Health noted that while unrestricted visiting for parents was common in 98 per cent of the 286 hospitals they surveyed, rather less than half restricted sibling visits and over 10 per cent restricted parental visiting to intensive care units. Although 94 per cent allowed rooming in by parents, only 50 per cent provided accommodation for this purpose.

A World Health Organization European publication (Stenbok 1986), looked at practice in 24 hospitals in nine countries 'chosen to be as representative as possible'. Eleven units had unrestricted visiting, nine allowed between 5 and 9 hours a day, one had 2 hours a day, two had 1 hour twice a week and one had none. Five out of the nine countries had no data on how many children were admitted to adult wards, an overall estimate was 65 per cent.

There have been big changes in Australia. The Association for the Welfare of Children in Hospital published a report in 1992 based on a 92.3 per cent response to a survey of over 300 hospitals. The majority of children were in separate paediatric wards, but there was a disturbing trend towards the closure of such units, apparently for financial reasons. Provision was offered to parents in most cases but only a small proportion actually told parents about this in advance.

There remains a not very hidden hazard: the cost for parents of children in hospital. Treatment may be free at the point of delivery in Britain and more or less free in many other countries but there remains the cost of visiting. In Australia the costs for parents of rooms and food varies widely from hospital to hospital and even in Britain where there are no such charges, there are fares to pay, time is lost from work, and alternative care may have to be arranged for siblings.

A survey of 13 different types of hospitals carried out in Britain by Action for Sick Children in the early 1990s found that 5.6 per cent of the families went into debt as a result of visiting costs, 12 per cent said that they would have nothing left at the end of the week to cover visiting costs, and 25.6 per cent said that they would have liked to have visited more often.

In 1984 the National Association for the Welfare of Children in Hospital published its charter, shown in Table 2.1. It demonstrates both how far we have come and how far there was still to go.

Similar statements on the rights of children and parents have been made by the Association for the Care of Children in Hospital in America, in 1980 and 1991, both of which had a powerful emphasis on privacy and respect for the individual.

While battles will continue, we can note that 7 years after the publication of the charter in Britain, the Department of Health issued guidance to all District Health Authorities which said 'A cardinal principle of hospital services for children is the complete ease of access to the child by his or her parents ... This is not a luxury.' (Department of Health 1991).

See also Chapter 8 on emotional factors.

Table 2.1   A charter for children in hospital

1. Children shall be admitted to hospital only if the care they require cannot be equally well provided at home or on a day basis.

2. Children in hospital shall have the right to have their parents with them at all times provided this is in the best interests of the child. Accommodation should therefore be offered to all parents and they should be helped and encouraged to stay. In order to share in the care of their child, parents should be fully informed about ward routine and their active participation encouraged.

3. Children and/or their parents shall have the right to information appropriate to age and understanding.

4. Children and/or their parents shall have the right to informed participation in all decisions involving their health care. Every child shall be protected from unnecessary medical treatment and steps taken to mitigate physical or emotional distress.

5. Children shall be treated with tact and understanding and at all times their privacy shall be respected.

6. Children shall enjoy the care of appropriately trained staff, fully aware of the physical and emotional needs of each age group.

7. Children shall be able to wear their own clothes and have their own personal possessions.

8. Children shall be in an environment furnished and equipped to meet their requirements, and which conforms to recognized standards of safety and supervision.

9. Children shall have full opportunity for play, recreation, and education suited to their age and condition.

National Association for the Welfare of Children in Hospital, London (now Action for Sick Children) (1984).

References

Bowlby, J. (1951). *Maternal care and mental health*. Monograph Series No 2. World Health Organization, Geneva.
Bowlby, J. (1965). *Child care and the growth of love*, (2nd edn). Penguin, Harmonsdworth.

Brandon, S. (1986). *Children in hospital*. National Association for the Welfare of Children in Hospital, London.

British Paediatric Association, National Association for the Welfare of Children in Hospital, National Association of Health Authorities, and Royal College of Nursing (1987). *Where are the children?* Brittish Paediatric Association, London.

Clarke, A.M. and Clarke, A.D.B. (1976). *Early experience: myth and evidence*. Open Books, London.

Department of Health and Social Security Committee on Child Health Services (1976). *Fit for the future*. (The Court Report.) HMSO, London.

Douglas, J.W.B. (1975). Early hospital admissions and later disturbances of behaviour and learning. *Developmental Medicine and Child Neurology*, **17**, 456–80.

Department of Health (1991). *Welfare of young children in hospital*. HMSO, London.

Doxiadis, S. (1970). Mothering and Frederik II. *Clinical Pediatrics*, **9**, 565–66.

Haslum, M.N. (1988). Length of preschool hospitalization, multiple admissions and later educational attainment and behaviour. *Child: Care, Health and Development*, **14**, 275–91.

Hinde, R.A. and Davies, L. (1972). Removing infant rhesus from mother for 13 days compared with removing mother from infant. *Journal of Child Psychology and Psychiatry*, **13**, 227–237.

Institute of Child Health and Society of Medical Officers of Health and Population (1954). *Report of the investigation committee*. London.

Ministry of Health (1959). *The welfare of children in hospital* (The Platt Report). HMSO, London.

Moncrieff, A. (1962). Visiting children in hospital. *Family Doctor*, **16**, 26–7.

Mrazek, D.A., Pollard, I.S., and Strunk, R.C. (1982). *Disturbed Emotional Development in Severely Asthmatic Preschool Children*. Paper presented at the 10th International Congress of the International Association for Child and Adolescent Psychiatry and Allied Professions, Dublin.

Pilowsky, T., Bassett, D.L., Begg M.W., and Thomas, P.G. (1982). Childhood hospitalization and chronic intractable pain in adults. *International Journal of Psychiatry in Medicine*, **12**, 75–84.

Prugh, D.G., Straub, E.M., Sands, H.H., Kirschbaum, R.M., and Lenihan, E.A. (1953). A study of the emotional reactions of children to hospitalization and illness. *American Journal of Orthopsychiatry*, **23**, 70–106.

Quinton, D. and Rutter, M. (1976). Early hospital admissions and later disturbances of behaviour: an attempted replication of Douglas's findings. *Developmental Medicine and Child Neurology*, **18**, 447–59.

Robertson, J. and Robertson, J. (1989). *Separation and the very young*. Free Association Books, London.

Sands, M.R. (1950). Visiting the child patient. *Nursing Times*, **8 July**.

Schaffer, H. and Callender, W.M. (1959). Psychologic effects of hospitalization in infancy. *Pediatrics*, **24**, 528–39.

Spitz, R.A. (1945). Hospitalism: an inquiry into the genesis of psychiatric conditions in early childhood. *The Psychoanalytic Study of the Child*, 1, 53–74.

Stenbok, E. (1986). *Care of children in hospital.* World Health Organisation Regional Office for Europe, Copenhagen.

Watson, J.B. (1928). *Psychological care of infant and child.* Allen & Unwin, London.

3

*Children in hospital today:
how many, what they do,
and who looks after them*

Some international comparisons of costs

It is not easy to draw direct comparisons between countries on expenditure on children's health and admissions to hospital partly because information is not recorded in a standard way. Crude data, examples of overall health expenditure as a percentage of gross national product, were given for 1986 by the Organization of Economic Cooperation and Development as follows: Canada 8.36, England and Wales 6.18, France 8.50, The Netherlands 8.33, Norway 6.82, and the USA 13 (American Academy of Pediatrics 1990).

Costs in Britain

Ten per cent of the expenditure on hospital and community health services in England and Wales is on children, of which hospitals account for approximately half. The pattern in Scotland is not widely different.

How many

The Audit Commission (1993) analysis of national data for the year 1990–1991 gives an estimate of 1 in 11 children and young people under the age of 19 years being 'admitted' per year but, as is discussed below, 'admitted' is a vague term.

One recent British estimate of hospital admissions is 10 per cent for the 0–4 year olds and 7 per cent for those aged between 5 and 15 years (Woodroffe and Glickman 1993), but it is extraordinarily difficult to say precisely either how many children are admitted as in-patients or whether this is an upward or downward trend.

Numbers of admissions

Up to 1985 returns of discharges from hospital in England and Wales were made to the Department of Health and Social Security. Between 1979 and 1985 there is a clear picture: more young children (0–4 years old) were admitted than in the older group (5–15 years old) and there was a steady trend upwards for all ages. Since then the age difference has remained in the same direction but a new system of returns has been introduced which makes comparisons difficult. Department of Health data for England for the year 1989–1990 record neither simple admissions nor discharges; they indicate instead that there were 764 000 finished consultant episode ordinary admissions, plus day cases, in the age group 0–4 years and 339 000 in the 5–15 year range (Department of Health 1993).

Taking these figures with the total child population one could arrive at an overall figure of 16 per cent, but some children will have been admitted more than once. Those with a chronic condition, asthma or cystic fibrosis, for example, are likely to be admitted more than once a year. In a study of a general hospital carried out in the early 1970s it was found that one-fifth of the children who were readmitted within 1 year were in hospital more than twice, usually up to five times (Cleary 1992). Another enquiry identified 'hospital veterans', children of 2 or 3 years old who had admissions well into double figures; one had been an in-patient 46 times by the time she was five years (Cleary 1992). When one realizes that between 10 and 15 per cent of children under 16 years of age in Britain suffer from chronic, long-term conditions (Eiser 1993), the need to take multiple admissions into account becomes evident.

In the United States there has been a slight shift in admissions when data from surveys published in 1981 and 1988 are compared: the latter figures showed 5 per cent fewer pre-schoolers and 4 per cent more adolescents (Association for the Care of Children's Health 1988). The most recent data from America indicates that there are approximately 3 000 000 admissions of children 18 years and under to all hospitals each year (4 per cent of all children). This does not mean, of course, that 3 000 000 different children are admitted, as noted above, there may be multiple admissions of the same patients.

There are relatively few admitted in the 15–19 years age group; the leading cause for those who are hospitalized is childbirth, with accidents and gunshot wounds coming second (Information from the National Association of Children's Hospitals and Related Institutions, USA, personal communication).

A statistical trap

There is another group, the so called 'hidden children', who come in for maybe a couple of hours for a test or the fitting of an appliance. They can form as much as 20 per cent of a ward's work-load (Thornes 1988).

Emergency admissions

In 1990–1991, 93 per cent of those children admitted to paediatrics and 68 per cent of those admitted to the main eight surgical specialties fell into this category (Audit Commission 1993). See also Chapter 16 on accident and emergency departments.

Length of stay and day cases

In Britain the mean length of stay has steadily declined, from 7 days in 1974 to 5 days in 1985 and to 4 days in 1989–90. (These figures are for 0–4 year olds in England and Wales; Department of Health 1991; Woodroffe *et al.* 1993.) It is unlikely that this pattern has changed since then and there has undoubtedly been a concomitant rise, dramatic in England and Wales at least, in the numbers of day cases. There were 68 423 in 1987–1988 and 123 381 in 1989–1990 (Department of Health 1991).

In the United States the overall mean length of stay in the 1988 survey was 7.1 days, with a striking difference between children in general hospitals (4.8 days) and those in specialist paediatric hospitals (10.4 days) (Association for the Care of Children's Health 1988). By 1993 the average had changed slightly to 6.09 days for patients in children's hospitals with paediatric residency programmes and 4.21 days in general hospitals without such programmes. Children whose health care is covered by Medicaid (the federal-state programme for the poor) stayed 1.2 days longer in children's hospitals (National Association of Children's Hospitals and Related Institutions, USA, personal communication).

Trends

Looking at previous admission figures may help to determine whether there has been a trend up or down but there are problems here, too. In 1987–1988 1 216 934 children aged 0–14 years were registered as having been admitted to hospital in England as in-patients (Department of Health 1991), but this is a questionable figure since it includes well babies and records that are admittedly deficient (Action for Sick Children 1991).

An upward trend is indicated in cohort studies, in which a group of children all born in the same period, usually a week, are followed up. A 1946 cohort reported that 18.5 per cent had been in hospital by the age of 5 years, compared with 25.5 per cent in a 1970 group (Golding and Haslum 1986).

Hill (1989) having looked at discharges from the Oxford region, concluded that despite the Platt and Court reports, children are now more likely to be admitted to hospital, although, as discussed below, the length of stay is shorter.

A report of the Department of Health and Social Security (1985) give further confirmation of an upward trend in both England and Wales. It should be noted, though, that the figures in this report are for discharges and, once again, some children will have been admitted more than once.

Where the children are cared for

Despite the recommendations of the Platt Report that children should not be nursed on adult wards, Department of Health data up to 1984 and the study by Hill (1989) suggest that fewer than half the children under 15 years in hospital in England and Wales were admitted to paediatric wards. By 1994 the picture had not improved dramatically; half the children admitted to English hospitals were not cared for by nurses qualified in the nursing of sick children and in Wales one-quarter were still admitted to adult wards (C. Hancock, BBC *Today Programme*, 12 April 1994).

As noted in Chapter 2, the picture in Australia is one in which the majority of children are cared for in paediatric rather than adult settings, but a 1992 report noted that although 95 per cent of general hospitals surveyed provided separate wards for children, at least 15 per cent of them placed children among other patients in a number of situations, for example on weekends or public holidays. Other hospitals reported that they place adults in children's wards when beds are vacant (Australia Association for the Welfare of Children in Hospital 1992).

Why they are admitted

Relying on mid-1980s' discharge rates we can say with some confidence, for England and Wales at least, that for children up to the age of 4 years diseases of the respiratory system were the most common cause, with the somewhat unsatisfactory category of 'signs, symptoms, and ill-defined conditions' coming second. For older children, the respiratory system accounts for most girls but injury and poisoning explain more boys' admissions.

Scottish data from records kept in 1990 go some way to confirm those from England and Wales in that respiratory disease and injury were the most common cause of admission of children aged 0–15 years (Common Services Agency 1992).

Findings from an Oxford study (Henderson *et al.* 1992) on children who had spent more than 5 days in hospital in that region, gave somewhat different figures from those given below in Tables 3.1–3.3, with congenital anomalies heading the list, followed by asthma, and then appendicitis. It should be remembered that these children had all been in hospital for longer than the average stay and the classification system used is different from that of the 1985 data set.

The data based on finished consultant episodes for 1990 corroborate the high rate of respiratory disorders and of accidents and injury found in previous years (see Table 3.1).

Another way of collecting data is to look at admissions by specialty. Of the patients aged 0–18 years in England and Wales, 1990–1991, the figures indicate that 44 per cent were to surgical specialties, 42 per cent went to paediatrics, and 14 per cent to others. Within the surgical group, ENT accounted for 12 per cent, followed by general surgery with 10 per cent and trauma and orthopaedics 9 per cent (Audit Commission 1993).

Diseases of the respiratory system are high on the list of reasons for the admission of young French children to hospital as well and the switch to disorders of the digestive system is marked in the 5–14 year olds, as is shown in Table 3.2.

Table 3.1 Discharge rates per 10 000 population in England and Wales for 0–4 year olds

Males
1. Diseases of the respiratory system	407.0
2. Signs, symptoms, and ill-defined conditions	282.9
3. Certain conditions originating in the perinatal period	209.2
4. Injury and poisoning	181.5
5. Diseases of the digestive system[a]	134.5
6. Congenital anomalies	129.2
7. Infectious and parasitic diseases	100.3
8. Diseases of the ear and mastoid process	65.7
9. Diseases of the genital organs	62.7
10. Hypoxia, birth asphyxia, and other respiratory conditions	57.5
11. Intestinal infections	49.5
12. Intercranial and internal injuries	48.5

Females
1. Diseases of the respiratory system	247.1
2. Signs, symptoms, and ill-defined conditions	222.8
3. Certain conditions originating in the perinatal period	176.6
4. Injury and poisoning	135.7
5. Infectious and parasitic diseases	88.3
6. Diseases of the digestive system[a]	80.6
7. Congenital anomalies	79.1
8. Diseases of the ear and mastoid process	47.5
9. Intestinal infections	41.8
10. Hypoxia, birth asphyxia, and other respiratory conditions	40.2
11. Intercranial and internal injuries	37.9
12. Poisoning and toxic effects	34.1

[a] excluding those of the oral cavity, salivary glands, and jaw.
Source: Department of Health and Social Security Office of Population Censuses and Surveys (1985). *Hospital in-patient enquiry*. Series MB4, no 26. HMSO, London.

The picture in the United States is not totally dissimilar to that seen in Britain. The main reasons for admission overall are respiratory conditions and congenital anomalies. Children with congenital or chronic conditions account for 65 per cent of patient days in children's hospitals. The leading causes of death in the first month of life (1989 data) were congenital anomalies such as Down's syndrome and spina bifida, followed by disorders related to prematurity and low birth weight, respiratory distress syndrome, and maternal complications of pregnancy. In the first year of life the leading causes of death were sudden

Children in Hospital

Table 3.2 Discharge rates per 10 000 population in England and Wales for 5–15 year olds

Males
1. Injury and poisoning		153.5
2. Diseases of the respiratory system		131.5
3. Signs, symptoms, and ill-defined conditions		93.9
4. Chronic diseases of tonsils and adenoids		59.3
5. Diseases of the ear and mastoid process		54.3
6. Intracranial and internal injuries		53.6
7. Fractures		51.3
8. Congenital anomalies		48.8
9. Diseases of the digestive system[a]		46.6
10. Diseases of the genital organs		39.5
11. Undescended testicle		25.2
12. Diseases of the musculoskeletal system and connective tissue		23.7

Females
1. Diseases of the respiratory system		111.7
2. Injury and poisoning		86.1
3. Signs, symptoms, and ill-defined conditions		78.6
4. Chronic diseases of tonsils and adenoids		69.4
5. Diseases of the ear and mastoid process		45.7
6. Diseases of the digestive system[a]		30.9
7. Fractures		30.5
8. Intracranial and internal injuries		25.5
9. Diseases of the musculoskeletal system and connective tissue		22.4
10. Congenital anomalies		20.1
11. Disorders of the eye and adnexa		14.6
12. Strabismus and other diseases of binocular eye movements		11.9

[a]excluding those of the oral cavity, salivary glands, and jaw.
Source: Department of Health and Social Security Office of Population Censuses and Surveys (1985). *Hospital in-patient enquiry*. Series MB4, no 26. HMSO, London.

infant death syndrome, congenital anomalies, preventable injuries, and pneumonia/influenza. After the age of 1 year, trauma kills more children than all diseases combined. For the 15–19 year age group homicide comes second after road traffic accidents (National Association of Children's Hospitals and Related Institutions, USA, personal communication).

Table 3.3 Finished consultant episode ordinary admissions plus day cases, year ending 31 March 1990, in England (expressed in thousands)

	0–4 years	5–14 years
Respiratory system	126	82
Injury and poisoning	52	77
Nervous system and sense organs	50	64
Digestive system	45	50
Genitourinary system	23	25
Neoplasms	8	13
Mental disorder	4	14
Circulatory system	2	1
Pregnancy, etc.	0	1
Other reasons	454	11
Total	764	339

From Department of Health (1993). *Health and personal social services statistics for England 1993 edition*. HMSO, London.

Table 3.4 Hospitalization of infants and children due to infectious and parasitic diseases and other diseases, France 1985–1987 (expressed in percentages)

	< 1 year	1–4 years	5–14 years
Infectious and parasitic diseases	10.4	9.2	4.4
Accidents and poisoning	4.3	21.8	26.8
Diseases of the respiratory system	12.0	19.8	8.7
Ill-defined symptoms and diseases	8.1	13.7	11.9
Diseases of the digestive system	5.9	6.8	15.3
Diseases of perinatal origin	32.0	0.0	0.0
Congenital malformations	9.0	5.2	6.6
Others	17.5	23.5	26.4

Manciaux, M. and Jesstin, C. (1990). Child health in 1990: the United States compared to Canada, England and Wales, France, The Netherlands and Norway. *Pediatrics*, **86**, (suppl.), 1025–127.
From Manciaux and Jesstin (1990).

What children do in hospital

It is a truism to say that to children hospitals are large, busy, confusing, and at times frightening places. Paediatric wards add to the confusion by the sheer level of activity that is often evident and the initial difficulty of sorting out who is who when doctors virtually never wear white coats, when some nurses' uniforms are a polo shirt and slacks, when some nurses wear their own clothes, and when it is not uncommon to use first names for everyone. (I can still remember hearing a 12 year old say, quite unself-consciously, 'I'll have to ask Judith.' Judith was the professor of haematology.)

But it does not take long to recognize a pattern, of activities and people. There is the ward routine, of treatments, of rounds, of play, of school, and meals and there is a recognizable pattern to the people. Most staff nowadays wear some kind of identification badge and even if these are not totally explicit it does not take long to realize that the chap in the open neck shirt is the consultant, the one with the beard is the chaplain, the tall dark-haired woman the sister, and so on. The more perceptive children also come to sense that despite the outward informality the hierarchical organization that has been in place since ever still exists.

A number of attempts have been made to monitor what children do in hospital and how they appear to feel. Twenty years ago, Hawthorn (1974) showed that the percentage of time children were alone was high and a number of them were characterized as 'miserable'. In 1980, a 9 year old American child wrote that she lost count of how many times she felt sad in hospital (Children of Bellevue Inc. 1980).

A recently published study has reported on the daily life of children in an eight-bedded room in a paediatric unit of three wards in Cardiff (Cleary 1992). It is discussed in detail here because the ordinary routine was seen to be similar to that found in many general hospitals. Direct, emergency, and planned admissions were received and there was a high patient turnover; only one child stayed in for the whole week of the observation period, while two were in for 6 days. The pressure to take patients was such that the ward often held ten beds instead of the planned eight. There was unrestricted visiting and one parent could stay overnight with any child.

Parents were expected to carry out basic care: washing, feeding, and toileting and some, having learned procedures that they would have to undertake once the child was discharged, nasogastric feeding being an example, would do them as well. The system of care by parents is relevant here. It has been described by Goodband and Jennings (1992) as 'A model for care of children in hospital in which the parents retain the responsibility for the care of their child, during hospitalisation, albeit with varying degrees of support.' The idea is discussed in detail in Chapter 21.

The hospital school catered mainly for children of primary age and there was a play specialist. The playroom was very small but the ward itself was spacious and there were opportunities to bring play to the children. It seemed, however, that play was restricted to occupying children, possibly because the very rapid turnover meant that it was difficult to get to know individuals.

Observations were carried out during 1 week between 6.15 a.m. and 11.30 p.m. No observations were made in the classroom, bathrooms, or toilets although a record was made of when children were known to be in school. During this week six boys and eight girls were admitted; the spread and range of their ages was wide, going from 21 months to 11 years.

The most likely place for children to be when on the ward was close to their own bed; this accounted for approximately half of all the observations of children who were not on or in bed. Of the remainder, nearly half were near the television, although not all children were watching the programme. The rest of the time was in someone else's bed space or in the open part of the ward. When children were off the ward they were most often (33 per cent) in the corridor just outside. This was more than just a passageway since many activities took place there: admission procedures, teaching rounds, discussions, and the dispensation of meals from the food trolley are just three examples. Next came the schoolroom at 11.6 per cent and a rather high 40.6 per cent of the off-the-ward time was at an unknown location.

One striking finding related to children's sleep. Although the timing of the observations, beginning before 7 a.m. and ending after 11 p.m., might have led to the expectation that all of them would be asleep for at least a couple of hours during this period, this was not so: in fewer than one-quarter of the observations made between 10 p.m. and 11.30 p.m. were they all in bed and asleep. The author notes that illness, plus the strangeness of the hospital and the absence of familiar rituals of story-telling, etc. could easily disturb sleep; several children who were settled early were found awake again after 8 p.m. What could not be observed was the depth of sleep each child went into. One could hypothesize that they tended to remain in the early stages rather more than they would have at home but this must be a speculation. There might, however, be an explanation here for some of the irritability that children show in hospital; certainly resident parents often say that they sleep badly.

Both children and parents often report that they are bored in hospital but the layout of this ward, plus the number of visitors and staff available, meant that the patients were seldom alone. The fact that it was an eight bedder rather than eight cubicles meant that if a child in distress had no one immediately available to provide comfort another parent in the absence of a nurse would offer support. For only 2 per cent of the observations were there no visitors and only 13 per cent reported no evident nurses. Three children who were on the ward for 3 or more days with a resident parent were alone during waking hours for less than 5 per cent of the observed times. The 11 year old was, appropriately perhaps, alone for 14 per cent of his waking time; others varied between 6 per cent and 30 per cent.

It is possible of course, that the older children would have preferred more time to themselves: 'awake and alone' tells us little, indeed, about the children's emotional state. A child who is reading or doing schoolwork may prefer to be left in peace; a child whose parent is sitting by the bedside but reading a newspaper may be comforted but may instead be lonely.

There was little overt crying, less than 2 per cent of the observations and then usually related to painful procedures, although it was sometimes noted that the children looked sad. There was a marked contrast with a babies' ward when the patients cried for one-fifth of the time they were awake.

Another characteristic finding, not surprising given the age range represented, was the variety of activities evident. In the author's words 'People without experience of children's wards tend to imagine neat rows of beds, each with a quiet occupant doing nothing more strenuous than a jigsaw puzzle, but this is not the case, nor would it be considered desirable.' At any one time children would be playing, eating, watching television, or just moving about.

Much of the time that children were away from their own beds was spent with other children, with wide individual variation. One 5 year old, a veteran well familiar with the ward routine, was often with others whereas a 4 year old was almost always alone or with his mother. It helps enormously if children can strike up a friendship as two did in this study. Some hospitals that cater for children who are admitted frequently often try to engineer admissions of friends simultaneously.

The list of activities followed included 'general running around and playing about' and more formal games and imaginative play. Dolls' prams and push chairs were used a great deal and jigsaws and board games and bricks and construction toys were also popular. Reading, even comics, was hardly ever recorded, a somewhat disturbing finding in accord with my own observations. It should be remembered that this study was conducted before the arrival in many hospital wards of computer games which older children now seem to get locked into for hours on end.

Much has been made of the number of different people children encounter in hospital. One study of a 2 year old (quoted in Cleary 1992) recorded that he was looked after by up to eight different nurses a day, with the weekly total being no fewer than 116 different nurses. On top came all the medical and ancillary staff as well. This, too, was looked at in the Cardiff study and patients' contacts were registered. The most frequent, 66 per cent, was with their parents, alone or with others. Nurses alone accounted for 11 per cent and nurses and others for 10 per cent. Doctors were only 1 per cent and doctors and others 2 per cent. Thus, although children came into contact with a wide range of people there was at least some stability provided by the very frequent presence of their parents.

Summarizing the conclusions of this study the author notes that there were certain key factors affecting children's lives in hospital. Three within-child variables were mobility, maturity, and language, all of which gave greater possibilities of control over the environment. External to children was the presence of a mediator, most often a parent but occasionally the play specialist.

Observations over another week or in a different hospital would yield data different from those reported here. Nevertheless, the overall conclusions on variability and the factors affecting children's lives can be generalized with some confidence.

References

Action for Sick Children (1991). *Statistics on children in hospital, keypoints series*. Action for Sick Children, London.

American Academy of Pediatrics (1990). Child health in 1990: the United States compared to Canada, England and Wales, France, The Netherlands and Norway. *Pediatrics*, **86**, (suppl.), 1025–1127.

Association for the Care of Children's Health (1988). *Directory of hospital psychosocial policies and programs.* Association for the Care of Children's Health, Washington, DC.

Australian Association for the Welfare of Children in Hospital (1992). *National survey report on psycho-social care of children (and families) in hospital.* Australian Association for the Welfare of Children in Hospital, New South Wales.

Children of Bellevue Inc. (1980). *Calendar.* The Child Life Program, Bellevue Hospital Center, New York.

Cleary, J. (1992). *Caring for children in hospital.* Scutari Press, London.

Common Services Agency (1992). *Hospital statistics, Scotland, 1991.* SHHD, Edinburgh.

Department of Health (1991). *Hospital episode summary tables, England, 1987–1988.* Government Statistical Service, London.

Department of Health (1993). *Health and personal social services statistics for England 1993 edition.* HMSO, London.

Department of Health and Social Security (1985). *Hospital in-patient enquiry.* Office of Population Censuses and Surveys, Series MB4, no 26. HMSO, London.

Eiser, C. (1993). *Growing up with a chronic disease.* Jessica Kingsley, London.

Golding, J. and Haslum, M. (1986). Hospital admissions. In *From birth to five*, (ed. N.R. Butler and J. Golding). Pergamon Press, Oxford.

Goodband, S. and Jennings, K. (1992). Parent care; a US experience in Indianapolis. In *Caring for children in hospital*, (ed. J. Cleary). Scutari Press, London.

Hawthorn, P.J. (1974). *Nurse—I want my mummy.* Study of Nursing Care Research Project, Series 1, No. 3. Royal College of Nursing, London.

Henderson, J., Goldacre, M.J., Fairweather, J.M., and Marcovitch, H. (1992). Conditions accounting for a substantial time spent in hospital in children aged 1–14 years. *Archives of Disease in Childhood*, **67**, 83–6.

Hill, A.M. (1989). Trends in paediatric medical admissions. *British Medical Journal*, **298**, 1479–83.

Thornes, R. (1988). *Where are the children? Caring for children in the Health Services.* Action for Sick Children, London.

Woodroffe, C. and Glickman, M. (1993). Trends in child health. *Children and Society*, **7**, 49–63.

Woodroffe, C., Glickman, M., Barker, M., and Power, C. (1993). *Children, teenagers and health: the key data.* Open University Press, Buckinghamshire.

4

What children understand about health, illness, and treatment

Introduction

Behind the many preparation programmes now offered in hospitals is the assumption that children can have some comprehension of what is being done to them and why. Behind the recent interest in the need to seek children's consent for investigations, treatment, and participation in research, is a similar assumption: that they can understand the implications of their condition.

For some time there has been an acknowledgement that adolescents might be asked to consent to treatment but younger children have until recently been dismissed as 'incompetents', small immature bodies being thought to contain small immature minds (Alderson 1993). This attitude has been changing in the past few years as is evident in the 1989 Children Act, which set out the need to seek consent from all children with sufficient understanding. The enormous potential impact of this legislation on the care of children in hospital has yet to be realized. (See Chapter 20 for a fuller discussion of the act.)

Deciding how much children can understand is not easy. One of the reasons this is such a perplexing topic is the limitation on young children's language skills; perhaps their ignorance is more apparent than real, as much to do with adults' inability accurately to discern what they think rather than a failure on their part.

We should also bear in mind that the world is a bewildering place for children; perhaps, like many adults, they use fantasy and magical thinking to reduce tension, resolve conflict, and fill in gaps in their knowledge (Peters 1978). If this view is correct, then we have to look at emotional as well as cognitive factors.

Before we look at how children understand their illnesses we should start at the beginning and see what they make of their bodies.

What children understand about their bodies

Very young children, the 3–4 year olds, probably understand very little. When they begin to draw a human in a recognizable form they leave the body out altogether, drawing the arms and legs coming from the head.

Early work on children's understanding of their bodies came from Schilder and Wechsler (1935) when they asked children to name what was inside them. The 4 year olds focused mainly on what they had eaten while older children, 11 years and over, gave more correct answers. This pattern has been repeated in almost every study carried out since then: young children's earliest concepts are psychological; breathing and thinking are perceived by pre-schoolers in terms of behaviours, what Carey (1985) has called 'intuitive psychology'. There is a steady increase in biological knowledge and a growing sophistication in children's ability to describe not only what is in the body but how it works (Crider 1981).

Nevertheless, many grow up with only a rather hazy idea of what is there and what goes on inside it. Pearson and Dudley (1982), for example, found that around 10 per cent of the 81 adults they studied thought that they had two livers.

A criticism of much of the methodology of the work that followed Schilder and Wechsler's (1935) pioneering study is that it constrains children. Many researchers have, for example, used the technique of asking children to draw body parts, often on to an outline and some are much better at drawing than others. Even those who are skilled may have problems in depicting in two dimensions something which is three-dimensional in actuality.

Despite these caveats, one can see, as was noted above, some developmental trends and some lessons can be learned in relation to work in hospital. Children certainly seem to learn more as they get older, hardly a surprising finding, but they also seem to learn about the inner parts of the body in a sequence: first comes the heart, then the brain and the stomach, and then the lungs. Knowledge of the kidneys, liver, and bladder is scant and the reproductive organs are rarely noted when children draw.

A Piagetian view has been put forward to explain the development of children's understanding of how the body works rather than just what is in it. Crider (1981) argued that 6 year olds have a global view of functioning with little clear understanding of the difference between the inside and outside. Later children can differentiate structures, for example, muscles are in the legs to help them bend. By 11 or 12 years children can organize their body into interdependent systems. Similar developmental trends were found by Johnson and Wellman (1982) when they reported that all the kindergarten children in their sample could locate the brain and all but one could give a reasonable account of its role in thinking. However, children of all ages seemed to restrict the role to mental activity; it was only adults who mentioned its function in motor behaviour. In work reported by Eiser and Patterson (1983) young children argued that only the mouth and teeth are involved in eating and only the legs and arms are required for swimming. The 6 year olds asserted that it is bones that make the legs move.

One might imagine that children who are sick will have been sensitized to gaining knowledge about those aspects of their bodies that relate to their condition. The evidence that exists supports this hypothesis: Eiser (1985) mentions that there is evidence for an accelerated and specific understanding in children with heart disease, cystic fibrosis, diabetes, and those undergoing surgery.

All this is relatively straightforward. The child's understanding of health and disease is much more complex.

Children's understanding of health

Most of the research in this area has looked at children's development of an awareness of health and how their ideas change over time. Thus, Rashkis (1965) found that children aged between 4 and 9 years old said that diet is an important aspect of health, as is protection by adults. Byler and Lewis (1969), in a study of 5000 children, found age-related shifts in the definitions of health from the younger children's simple, behaviourally rooted ideas ('isn't too fat or too skinny') to more detailed answers. Similar results were found by Natapoff (1978).

Eiser *et al.* (1983) studied 80 children aged 6–11 years and found that taking exercise and being energetic were the most common ways of defining health for all ages combined. Some older children mentioned resistance to infection.

Cultural and environmental factors must play some part in determining what children regard as health. Zinkin (personal communication 1994) noted an unusual response, from a child in Nicaragua: 'to be healthy you have to have a tranquil conscience'.

Healthy children's understanding about illness

Two themes run through the literature: the way in which children's thinking in this area progresses through a number of stages and the notion that illness is a punishment for wrong doing.

Stages of understanding

Nagy (1951) put forward the idea that children's ideas develop in stages.

1. Under 6 years they see cause and effect contiguous in time.

2. At 6–7 years illness is caused by an unspecified infection.

3. At 8–10 years illness is caused by microorganisms.

4. At 11–12 years different illnesses are caused by different organisms.

A review of the literature by Bibace and Walsh (1981) concluded that developmental considerations can help us understand children's theories. The younger the child the more likely he or she is to produce a simple, concrete explanation, poorly organized in terms of process, employing few categories to define health and illness. Age brings complexity and sophistication of thinking.

These authors looked to Piaget to provide a theoretical framework within which to explain the shifts from the concrete to the abstract. Their own study, published in 1980, supported this view. They interviewed 72 children aged 4–11 years in order to arrive at a concept of illness. Sample questions were as follows.

1. Were you ever sick?

2. How did you get sick?

3. How did you get better?

4. What is a heart attack?

5. Why do people get a heart attack?

6. What are germs?

7. What do they look like?

8. Can you draw germs?

9. Where do they come from?

When answers were coded they were seen to fall into three groups, fitting Piaget's stages of cognitive development. The first was pre-logical (people get colds from trees, from outside, when someone else gets near them). The second is concrete-logical when children can distinguish between the internal and the external (people get colds when they are outside without a hat ... your head would get cold ... the cold would touch it and then it would go all over your body). This illustrates another hurdle for English-speaking children: the possible confusion between cold referring to the temperature and cold meaning an illness.

The third stage is formal-logical when the source of the illness is perceived to be within the body even though an external agent may be the actual cause.

A later review by Burbach and Peterson (1986) concluded that although there are methodological weaknesses in many studies, most data 'appear to suggest that children's concepts of illness do evolve in a systematic and predictable sequence consistent with Piaget's theory of cognitive development'. This conclusion is not without its critics, however. Eiser *et al.* (1990) looked at what children's stories can tell us about illness, with children aged 5 and 8 years, and concluded that their experience was a better explanation for the understanding than stage theory. This is discussed further below in the section on sick children's understanding.

Immanent justice

Some studies carried out since the 1940s have concluded that many children blame themselves for their illness, seeing their symptoms and/or their treatment as a form of punishment for wrong doing. The phrase 'immanent justice' is often used to sum up this belief: you do something wrong and wham—you break your leg or catch cold or worse. An example is the work of Gellert (1961) who found that the majority of her 30 healthy children aged 4–16 years blamed human agents or human actions for illness.

This is not altogether surprising. We all of us, adults as well as children, need to make sense of our world, to fit the new and the strange into a known context. So if we are suddenly ill and if no-one has given any other explanation, then we have to fill the vacuum that is uncertainty and one ready explanation is blame. It is not a new idea. When seventeenth-century Ralph Josselin's son died he regarded it as a punishment from God for his excessive fondness for playing chess

(Macfarlane 1970). Puritans, on both sides of the Atlantic, 'clearly believed that God held all members of the nuclear family as hostages for the good behaviour of any one of them' (Stone 1977).

This explanation will be all the more powerful if children have recently hurt themselves while doing something they were warned not to. It will be superpowerful if they come from families where medical staff are held up as avengers: 'If you don't go to bed at once I'll call that nurse to give you another injection.'

Since this early work there has been a shift away from such an emphasis on children using the notion of immanent justice, possibly because there is much more care taken now to explain illness to them, possibly because parents are more sophisticated than they were a generation ago. Instead a wide range of interpretations is looked to, with a much greater realization that developmental factors come into play. Writing in America, Brodie (1974) found that only 25 per cent of the children studied believed that boys and girls who misbehave get sick more often that those who are good; and recent work on the causes of pain, discussed in Chapter 9, has tended not to give such prominence to immanent justice.

A good example of the wide range of causes invoked comes in a study by Kister and Patterson (1980). They asked questions of 60 children at four age levels. Younger children were, indeed, more likely to see immanent justice as an explanation for both contagious and non-contagious illnesses and accidents and children of all ages saw a blame element in illness as opposed to accidents. But the older they were, the more they seemed able to understand that immanent justice is a poor reason for illness.

One rather worrying study, worrying if it were to be generally true, found that at least some pre-school children in America thought that hospital was a place that made people ill (Redpath and Rogers 1984). This harks back to the views of many adults a couple of generations ago, when they perceived that going to hospital was a sure step towards death.

Sick children's ideas about illness

Stages of thinking

A Piagetian progression has been noted similar to that found in healthy children. There is a reported shift from global, magical, undifferentiated thinking ('You get sick from kissing old people and women') to a more sophisticated awareness of principles ('illness is caused by catching germs from other people') (Simeonsson *et al.* 1979; Perrin and Gerrity 1981; Brewster 1982).

There has, however, been a move to question Piagetian theories in the last few years. Eiser (1989) argued in support of alternative theories which give greater emphasis to the role of experience. Eiser's (1989) criticism of stage theories is more than academic: she is unhappy with the assumption that we should use explanations of bodily functions based on concrete everyday experiences, the soldiers of chemotherapy who fight the enemy bad cells, for example. It is not clear to her that such analogies are always helpful, for young children may take them literally.

Alderson (1993) took up the questioning of Piaget. Commenting on the children in her study, aged 8–15 years, she concludes that they clearly did not realize how incompetent they were supposed to be. She goes on to give examples of quite sophisticated thinking in this age group, concluding that 'the popularity of Piaget's theories has outlasted their credibility perhaps because they are convenient to the most powerful group of all, adults'.

Immanent justice and the sick child

Although Gellert (1961) noted healthy children were more likely to explain illness in terms of human action or default than those who were sick, there is a certain body of evidence, reviewed by Peters (1978) to suggest that sick children do tend to blame human wrong doing for illness.

My own experience suggests that at least in recent years such blaming is relatively rare, but it happens: a teenage girl with cancer said, a couple of days before she died, 'I want to go to heaven for one day to ask God what I have done to make me suffer so much.'

Children's perceptions of the intent of treatment

If children do think that they are ill because they have been naughty then it is likely to follow that they perceive treatment as a punishment. Much of the literature to support this view is based on a psychoanalytic standpoint; see Peters (1978) with the not surprising conclusion that it is the younger children who tend in this direction. Brazelton *et al.* (1953) found that some children saw treatments used by the hospital staff as a means of controlling the patients.

Conclusion

Bringing all this into a practical perspective, Eiser (1985) concludes that young children's misconceptions about disease might lead to conflict in their accepting treatment: 'There can surely be no finer argument for better preparation and information about disease to be made available for the young chronically sick child.' She goes on to elaborate the needs to tailor this preparation to the cognitive level of the child in question, a point taken up in Chapter 7.

See also Chapter 10 for a discussion of children's understanding of death and heaven.

References

Alderson, P. (1993). *Children's consent to surgery*. Open University Press, Buckingham.

Bibace, R. and Walsh, M.E. (1981). Children's conceptions of illness. In *New directions for child development: no 14. Children's conceptions of health, illness and bodily functions*, (ed. R. Bibace and M.E. Walsh). Jossey-Bass, San Francisco.

Brazelton, T.B., Holder, R., and Talbot, B. (1953). Emotional aspects of rheumatic fever in children. *The Journal of Pediatrics*, LXIII, 339–58.

Brewster, A.B. (1982). Chronically ill hospitalized children's concepts of their illness. *Pediatrics*, **69**, 355–62.

Brodie, B. (1974). Views of healthy children towards illness. *American Journal of Public Health*, **64**, 1156–9.

Burbach, D.J. and Peterson, L. (1986). Children's concepts of physical illness: a review and critique of the cognitive–development literature. *Health Psychology*, **5**, 307–25.

Byler, R. and Lewis, G. (1969). *Teach us what we want to know*. Mental Health Materials Center, New York.

Carey, S. (1985). *Conceptual change in childhood*. The MIT Press, Cambridge, MA.

Crider, C. (1981). Children's concepts of the body interior. In *New directions for child development: no 14. Children's conceptions of health, illness and bodily functions*, (ed. R. Bibace and M.E. Walsh). Jossey-Bass, San Francisco.

Eiser, C. (1985). *The psychology of childhood illness*. Springer-Verlag, New York.

Eiser, C. (1989). Children's concepts of illness: towards an alternative to the 'stage' approach. *Psychology and Health*, **3**, 93–101.

Eiser, C. and Patterson, D. (1983). Slugs and snails and puppy-dog tails: children's ideas about the insides of their bodies. *Child: Care, Health and Development*, 9, 233–40.

Eiser, C., Patterson, D., and Eiser, J.R. (1983). Children's knowledge of health and illness: implications for health education. *Child: Care, Health and Development*, 9, 285–92.

Eiser, C., Eiser, R., Lang, J., and Mattock, A. (1990). What children's stories tell us about their understanding of illness. *Early Child Development and Care*, 57, 1–7.

Gellert, E. (1961). *Children's beliefs about bodily illness*. Paper presented at the American Psychological Association, 1 September.

Johnson, C.N. and Wellman, H.M. (1982). Children's developing conceptions of the mind and brain. *Child Development*, 53, 222–34.

Kister, M.C. and Patterson, C.J. (1980). Children's conceptions of the causes of illness: understanding of contagion and the use of immanent justice. *Child Development*, 51, 839–46.

Macfarlane, A. (1970). *Family life of Ralph Josselin*. The University Press, Cambridge.

Nagy, M.H. (1951). Children's ideas of the origin of illness. *Health Education Journal*, IX, 6–12.

Natapoff, J. (1978). Children's views of health. *American Journal of Public Health*, 68, 995–1000.

Perrin, E.C. and Gerrity, P.S. (1981). There's a demon in your belly: children's understanding of illness. *Pediatrics*, 67, 841–9.

Peters, B.M. (1978). School-aged children's beliefs about causality of illness: a review of the literature. *Maternal Child Nursing*, 7, 143–54.

Pearson, J. and Dudley, H.A.F. (1982). Bodily perceptions in surgical patients. *British Medical Journal*, 284, 1545–6.

Rashkis, S. (1965). Child's understanding of health. *Archives of General Psychiatry*, XII, 10–17.

Redpath, C.C. and Rogers, C.R. (1984). Healthy young children's concepts of hospitals, medical personnel, operations and illness. *Journal of Pediatric Psychology*, 9, 29–40.

Schilder, P. and Wechsler, D. (1935). What do children know about the interior of the body? *International Journal of Psychoanalysis*, 16, 345–50.

Simeonsson, R., Buckley, L., and Monson, L. (1979). Conceptions of illness causality in hospitalized children. *Journal of Pediatric Psychology*, 4, 77–84.

Stone, L. (1977). *The family, sex and marriage*. Weidenfeld and Nicolson, London.

5

Communicating with children and parents

Introduction

Communication between a hospital and family begins the moment the appointment letter is received: is it warm or couched impersonally? Is there a *Welcome to hospital* booklet enclosed, giving basic information about everyday routines that can be expected? On arrival at the hospital, are the main entrance and all other parts of the building well signposted? When patients arrive on a ward or in an out-patient department, are they met with blank stares or is it clear that they are expected? (One hospital I have heard of puts the names of the expected children over their beds before they arrive.)

Communication must be two way. The provision of an opportunity for patients and their families to ask when they do not know, to say what they mean, and to request what they need is essential. A climate which encourages even the most shy to make enquiries, to make suggestions, or to put in a request, is one which is in itself a great aid to recovery. A tiny example, or at least it seemed to *us*, was when a 9 year old girl in intensive care, who had been distressed, was able to ask if she could wear knickers under her nightie in bed. Of course she could; she was much happier once she did, but she had to ask.

Taking a somewhat arbitrary distinction, communication can be seen to serve two functions, related to facts and feelings.

Communicating factual information

'Children and/or their parents shall have the right to information appropriate to their age and understanding' (Charter of the National Association for the Welfare of Children in Hospital).

Many times parents have said that the first thing they wanted when they came to hospital was information. 'I didn't want sympathy, I wanted facts, delivered with brisk optimism', as one father put it. So once families are part of the hospital system the first need is to communicate something of the medical understanding of the child's condition and something of the possible plans for the immediate future. The extent to which the child will be involved in this is discussed in Chapter 20 in the section on informed consent.

The pitfalls of information giving are now well known: parents and patients, whatever their age, frequently do not take in what they have been told and may not even remember having been told anything, due partly to raised anxiety. The solutions are also reasonably well known: have someone else sitting in on the interview so that information can be repeated, perhaps several times, use written material to back up what has been said, and tape record the sessions.

Even if children are not directly part of the process of decision making about their treatment they can still be part of the system. One of the main aims of encouraging communication with children is to help them reduce their anxiety. It is hard for adults to appreciate not only how anxious children can be but also what misapprehensions they may have which fuel worries.

Children with leukaemia, knowing their blood count is low, can be worried when they have a finger prick for this is taking away precious blood which is, to them, already low.

Children with a degenerative disease may invoke all manner of fantasies to explain their reduced performance.

At a more immediate level we need to communicate with children in order to let them know what is happening to them and, perhaps even more important, what is going to happen. This is taken up further in Chapter 7 on preparation.

Cultural factors come in here. It is all very well when everyone shares the same value system; it may be quite different if the family come from a culture where authority is revered, where it would be unthinkable for a child to be given medical information, even more unthinkable for a child to question an adult's wishes, and off the graph for anyone to contradict the views of a doctor. Do we follow what we think is the right course even if this contravenes the belief system of the people we are talking to? There is no easy answer.

Communicating feelings

We need also to bring children into the discussions on their care, if for no other reason than to acknowledge that they are there, as human beings. The front page of the November 1993 issue of '*Cascade*', the journal of Action for Sick Children, carried the following from A.B., aged 11 years:

What do you see when you're looking at me?
Simply the girl in bed three?
But look at me.

A person
insecure and apprehensive as doctors whirl by.
A person.
With thoughts and feelings ... a heart.

What do you see when you're looking at me?
Simply the girl in bed three?

But I am a person who longs to rollerskate,
dance and skip ...
to be well again.

So, as I lie here, calm and still,
as I do as you wish,
as I eat at your will,

study me closely as you're rushed off your feet.
You're busy on night shift, no time for a seat.
An unusual case, a case to confirm.
No, I'm one of many,
if only you'd learn.

So open your eyes, doctor,
open and see,
not a fascinating case.

Look more closely.
Try to see me.

At this level communication is central to emotional support. Hilton Davis, a London psychologist, sees what he calls 'facilitative communication' as the means to help people help themselves. 'You may not take away the pain, but your respectful presence may make the anguish more tolerable. If nothing else, you can make people feel good about themselves and therefore more competent and effective, no matter what the problem' (Davis 1993).

Basic skills

The basic skills of communication are often evident to people observing an interchange but less obvious to those engaged in it. The initial task is to gain the others' confidence. This partly depends on personalities, partly on the perception of roles. A nurse or a doctor has a relatively easy time because they have clearly defined roles; others are likely to find the initial contact harder due to suspicion on the part of the child or parent. Titles easily get in the way: a psychologist or psychiatrist is often regarded as one who is 'wheeled in for the loonies' and many parents feel their pride is attacked when approached by a social worker. One group of parents with whom I worked decided that none of the conventional labels for psychosocial staff was adequate; they suggested that the term 'support worker' would be more appropriate.

Whatever the name given by the children or their parents, there comes the hurdle of the first session. The aim is to build up trust not only in the child but in the parents as well. There are a number of points of technique here.

The first is a consideration of the importance of the first few seconds, of the need to show respect for the people we are to be with. (How many professionals knock on a child's door before going into the cubicle or room?) Who is to be spoken to first? Young, shy children often prefer that they are not addressed directly for a few minutes, while older ones resent being left out. The choice of seating is important as well. If people are seen in the staff member's room it helps put them at their ease to indicate where they might sit, although sometimes it is instructive to watch their unaided choices. Wherever it may be, there should be an open space between the child and the person communicating and it is less threatening if the adult is more or less at the same height as the child.

I like to explain that I am a psychologist; I usually say 'the ward psychologist' to imply that all wards/units in my hospital have someone like me and to explain that my role is to do with how people think and feel.

What personal name one uses is not as easy as it may seem. The trend is increasingly for everyone to use first names and while children are usually comfortable with this their parents may not be, especially if they come from a culture which is on the formal side. It is harder dealing with how much to reveal of oneself. Children and adults have asked if I am married, if I have children. Sometimes I am asked if I have children with problems of any kind, sometimes children ask me about my religious beliefs. A large proportion of professionals duck all such questions; I tend towards the view that to refuse to answer at all is arrogant and counter-productive. What is critical is that each person comes to a carefully thought response.

The standard next step after the introductions is to talk about something emotionally neutral but relevant to the child. It helps, for example, to spend a little time looking around at the way the child has decorated the cubicle or bed area and then to embark on a brief conversation about their favourite pop star/football team or whoever is evident. If all else fails one can always talk about hospital food. But this can be rather false, embarrassing the adults and puzzling the child. If there is a clear agenda, for example if the child has a well-known fear of needles, I like to go straight into that topic fairly quickly. Beating about the bush can easily make children even more suspicious.

Maureen Hitcham, a social worker at the Royal Victoria Infirmary in Newcastle upon Tyne, prefers a more structured approach to her first interview and uses a sentence completion task with children, with items like 'I am the kind of person ...' or 'It seems difficult ...'. This gives her a baseline from which to work and with which to compare later responses to the same task.

Far too often communication is discussed in terms of a one-way flow, yet if we are really aiming to make others feel good about themselves we must not only listen to them but, especially when we are with children, we must let them know that we are receptive to what they have to say. We need to get across the message that we are able and willing to attend to them and that we are not going to judge them by what they say. I worked once with a 7 year old boy who was having panic attacks; wherever he was he wanted to be somewhere else and when in a panic would rush from one room to another. We were getting nowhere in therapy until one day he said that he wanted to say something that he thought I might find strange. I assured him that he could say anything he liked and he went on to say that the feeling he had when in a panic was like the one he had experienced when he had an operation at the age of 3 years. He described how, although he had received an anaesthetic, he felt the tube going down his throat. He thought this was a mad thing to say, but had to say it. Discussions with medical colleagues a few days later enabled me to tell him that in very, very, rare cases people can feel as he remembered. His panic attacks stopped.

Related to this assurance that we are listening in a non-judgemental way and part of the building of trust is the need, sometimes, to explain the confidential nature of a conversation. This is not difficult but if it is to be done it should be discussed as early as possible in the interaction.

Related also to the assurance that we are listening is the repertoire of non-verbal cues that come into play. Not letting our gaze wander, nodding occasionally, smiling at appropriate moments, not being distracted by others or by the telephone, all help to convey the essential message, 'I am attending to you; you are important to me.' We need to be able to show that we are attending to the child by our gaze, by our body language, by our facial expression, and by sharing a language.

Richman (1993) has worked extensively with children traumatized by civil war and has written on communicating with them. She has a number of excellent practical suggestions for workers in this field, one of which is to try to remember someone who has been a good listener to oneself. What were the characteristics of that person that made him or her so helpful?

Another component to the process is interpreting. Here we run into all sorts of problems due to the difficulty both of the word and of the act. I am not for a moment advocating that staff who have not been trained to do so should attempt to interpret inner meanings from what children say or do. Nevertheless, if we try to understand what children seem to be expressing at the level of the here and now we can help a great deal. The child who rounds on his or her mother, spitting, 'I hate you' is, in nine cases out of ten, expressing a hatred of the fact that the all powerful parent could not prevent the illness and now cannot organize a cure. It is likely to help if both parent and child can explore this interpretation.

Helping the communication of feelings

Oral communication can take many forms on a continuum from the direct to the oblique. The most direct question I have put to a patient was simple, 'When do you think you're going to die?' (I knew him very well.) The reply was, 'In about a week' which turned out to be true and allowed a free and useful discussion of the implications of his death. A more oblique example came from a girl who, in early December, told her parents not to bother to buy her any Christmas presents.

If we are using spoken language we should try to use open rather than closed questions. Closed questions are those that invite an answer 'yes' or 'no' or which are best answered factually. 'What is your name?' is a closed question, as is 'Did you have a good time in school today?' These can be compared with, 'What happened next?' or 'Tell me about your family.'

Many children are reluctant to talk about themselves but will listen intently when another child is talking, seeming to gain much from the realization that they are not unique. It is not always possible to find the right other child to have a conversation with but puppets can come in here. The puppet who 'talks' to the adult, saying how worried he is about his illness and how he wishes he could give all the doctors a needle every day, can do wonders.

Young children cannot use verbal language with sufficient facility to express all their emotions and for many play is the only available means of communication. Some play out fantasies, play at procedures (before and after), and play through anger. Children who have been stressed in hospital may suffer from a post-traumatic stress disorder to some degree and will need compulsively to relive the experience in some symbolic form or by talking about it. Incidentally, it is worth watching for the child who seems driven to play out or draw the same episode repeatedly since this is likely to indicate a need to talk about the experience.

Sometimes it is enough simply to observe free play, sometimes it is necessary to wait one's moment before probing. Roger was just 5 years old. The ward staff were concerned because he seemed so pre-occupied with his illness. He refused to draw or to tell stories for me so games of his choice were played on several occasions. One evening, when his mother had gone for supper, he said he wanted to play with Lego. He built a room which he announced was a laboratory. This led on to an imaginary conversation about patients whose blood was being tested in the laboratory and that led on in turn to a discussion of the implications of their illness if treatment were unsuccessful. He said, flatly, that they would die. Here, at last was an opportunity to ask him outright if he thought he was going to die.

He said sadly that he thought he would but added that he did not want to. Once that point had been reached we were able to take up his anxieties further.

Drawing and painting, both easily accessible to most children, provide both opportunities and pitfalls. As in play children can communicate specific messages. Christopher, 6 years old when he died, drew a small boat tossed in a storm, supported by two large whales. In an unpublished study carried out at Great Ormond Street Hospital, sick children were asked to draw themselves in hospital and siblings were asked to draw their brother or sister. There was a striking difference between the two sets of pictures: siblings drew a child surrounded by staff and visitors, while the sick children drew themselves in bed, isolated. More striking was another, also unpublished, study carried out by Stephens-Parker (1990). She compared the use of colour in pictures drawn by children with leukaemia compared to those attending a dental department and a healthy comparison group. There was a highly significant difference, with the sick children using far fewer colours.

A discussion of a system of scoring family drawings is given in Spinetta and Deasy-Spinetta (1981). This scoring system is not to be confused with the rather more vague interpretation of drawings which reads all sorts of meanings into the picture. As mentioned above, interpretation is not to be undertaken lightly, for it can lead into traps: one author has suggested that children's souls are aware of the time of their impending death and that they portray this in their pictures. So a tree with seven leaves predicts death in 7 days. This is scientifically worthless and psychologically preposterous.

One technique I have found useful to help parents express their feelings is to encourage them to distinguish between what they think intellectually and what they feel. I usually ask them to tell me what they think in their heads and in their guts. This has a two-fold message: one is that it is permissable to have two levels of thought, the other that both can be discussed.

Structured activities for children

Games can be a great help. The 'All About Me' game produced by Barnado's (available from Being Yourself, address given at the end of this chapter) enables children and adults to communicate about all sorts of feelings in a supportive, non-threatening way. It consists of an attractive board, with counters and dice and a set of cards with questions on them that the people taking part take turns to answer.

Other materials available from the same address include the *Drawing out feelings* series, designed to help children cope with feelings resulting from loss and change. They have some excellent ideas but within one book tend to switch developmental levels in a way that leads to the suggestion that bits of them should be used rather than the complete book.

'Life story' books can help facilitate communication at particularly difficult times. The basic idea is to record key elements in a person's life in such a way that feelings can be expressed, directly or indirectly, in a way that feels safe. Their complexity and their content will depend on the child. They may consist simply of episodes or people in the immediate present. On the other hand, there may be a family tree, with photographs of parents and grandparents, aunts and uncles, followed by an account of earliest memories, then recollections of the first illness, the first admission to hospital, and so on.

One girl in hospital, gravely ill, had lost her mother in tragic circumstances. Other members of her family could not bring themselves to tell her that her mother was dead, yet they could not bring themselves to lie to her either so the mother was never mentioned. The girl made a life story book starting with pictures of all the ward staff. She was then encouraged to start a new section to include all the people she had known who had died. Finally she was given photographs of her family. When her mother's picture came up she looked at it sadly and put it in the page with the other dead relatives.

A variant on life story books has been devised by Rebekah Lwin, a psychologist at Great Ormond Street who works with children in isolation. She encourages children in hospital and at home to keep their own scrap books-cum-diaries. As well as recording everyday events they can include photographs of visitors, comments from people around, souvenirs of certain incidents, and so on. Then when the children go home there can be a sharing of what has been happening to everyone in the period of absence.

Maureen Hitcham, mentioned above, has produced a first-rate video on communicating with parents and siblings about children with cancer and has written a handbook to go with it containing a range of activities to help children explore thoughts and feelings. As she has put it, 'Inside every child there is a story to be told'.

Communicating with parents

Although much of what has been written above refers to parents as well as children, there are some areas distinct to them, highlighted in the Audit Commission (1993) report. Their conclusion is simply that staff do not give enough time to the topic. In a survey of 48 families, many parents reported that they felt their role on the ward was unclear and that their own knowledge of their children was often ignored. What seemed to come out most explicitly from the survey was the lack of a clearly stated policy on parental involvement in care. This is the starting point of the commission's proposals for improvement, outlined below.

Improving communication with parents

First there should be a clear management focus, with written policies, for child and family-centred care. This policy should include the following.

1. The involvement of the child's family in care.

2. The nomination of a 'named nurse' for each child. This nurse is responsible for the care of each child for the duration of the stay, providing a link with others during the admission and afterwards. Out-patient departments should try to organize rotas so that the nurses see the same families each time they attend.

3. Written information which includes policies specific to individual departments, the facilities and services offered in the hospital, details about the management of individual conditions and procedures, and contact points for more information.

4. A family information service open most of the day containing comprehensive information about the hospital and related organizations, for example, self-help groups.

A policy such as this can be implemented at relatively little cost.

References

Audit Commission (1993). *Children first: a study of hospital services.* National Health Service Report No 7. HMSO, London.

Davis, H. (1993). *Counselling parents of children with chronic illness or disability*. British Psychological Society, Leicester.

Spinetta, J.J. and Deasy-Spinetta, P. (ed.) (1981). *Living with childhood cancer*. Mosby, St Louis.

Stephens-Parker, S. (1990). Unpublished dissertation. Psychology Department, University of East London.

Richman, N. (1993). *Communicating with children*. Save the Children, London.

Being Yourself, 73 Liverpool Road, Deal, Kent CT14 7NN, UK.

The video referred to is entitled *Over the Rainbow* and is obtainable from Maureen Hitcham, Malcolm Sergeant Social Worker, The Royal Victoria Infirmary, Newcastle on Tyne.

6

Play

The food and drink of mental growth, play, is an essential requirement for a child's well-being and development.

Deprived of play the child is a prisoner, shut off from all that makes life real and meaningful. Play is not merely a means of learning the skills of daily living. The impulse to create and achieve, working through play, allows the child to grow in body and mind ... Play is one of the ways in which a child may develop a capacity to deal with the stresses and strains of life as they press upon him. It acts, too, as a safety valve, allowing him to relive and often come to terms with fears and anxieties which have become overwhelming. Organisation Mondiale pour l'Education Préscolaire (1966).

All children should have access to good quality safe and affordable play opportunities, with supervision provided where appropriate, in accordance with age and need. (National Children's Bureau 1992).

Why children play

Early theories of play saw it as a means of working off surplus energy (Spencer 1898) or a way of providing early training in and practice of the skills to be required in adult life (Groos 1898, 1901). Rather more fancifully, play was seen as a recapitulation of the life styles and behaviour of our ancestors (Garvey 1977).

Piaget spent his life exploring how children come to understand their world. His was a stage-related theory and in it play goes along with other activities, i.e. there is first practice play, then symbolic play, and after that rule-bound play. He saw play as a means by which children assimilate information; it helps them to fit experience into a framework of understanding that has already been built up. He also saw it as providing a child with a unique individual experience and language to express feelings, thus laying the foundations of normal emotional development (Piaget 1951).

Huizinga (1955) emphasized the part that play has in helping children to acquire cultural roles and behaviour and to develop interpersonal relationships.

The psychodynamic approach focused much more on emotional development than Piaget had. Freud's original ideas of play as either an unconscious expression of a painful memory or desire or a re-enactment of a pleasant experience were developed by his daughter Anna (Freud 1936). Along with Klein (1929) she developed a therapeutic technique, play therapy, in which children's free play replaced the verbal free-association technique used in adult psychoanalysis. It is, incidentally, of the utmost importance to distinguish play therapy conducted by a trained child psychotherapist from free play in hospital. The former involves a therapist interpreting play to a disturbed child, while the latter involves a play specialist understanding a child's psychological needs, with the basic assumption of play in hospital being that children show normal reactions to abnormal situations, not that they are emotionally disturbed in the more general sense.

Erikson (1963) was also concerned with emotional distress, seeing play as a way of dealing with anxiety, enabling children to make up for defects, sufferings, and frustrations, 'The most natural auto-therapeutic measure childhood affords.'

He also put forward the view that through play children can create worlds in which they are free to try out new roles and master new situations and in so doing to form their own identity.

Highly pertinent to hospital play is the work of Herron and Sutton-Smith (1971) who argued that play helps children exercise control, blending reality with fantasy to create a scenario in which they are in charge, often used at a time when in fact they have none. Playing at doctors and nurses is an obvious and often observed example.

Stages and types of play

Although the rigid stage approach associated with Piaget is now no longer accepted by many developmental psychologists, it is helpful to consider play in certain crude stages. Babies and children up to the age of approximately 18 months to 2 years play on their own. They like to have a familiar adult nearby but do not interact in play. Activity is intense, in short bursts, and repetition becomes important. The next stage is so-called parallel play when children like to be alongside each other, frequently looking to see what the other is doing but interacting only briefly. Finally, around the ages of 3 dren play with others, in pairs or small groups.

Types of play

Some will no doubt argue that it is artificial to try to dissect children's play; all we should do is accept that play is play. On the other hand, there are times when some classification helps to understand why children behave as they do, what they do at certain times of their stay in hospital. Activities have been described as: exploratory play, energetic play, skilful play, social play, creative play, problem-solving play, destructive play, and hobbies.

A number of books on hospital play carry examples of all the above and give also ideas for adapting the hospital situation to encourage a wide range of activities (Harvey and Hales-Tooke 1972; Weller 1980; Jolly 1981).

Play in hospital

In a recently published report (Save the Children 1989), five functions of play in hospital were noted.

Aiding normality

There are two aspects here. One is that play is a normalizing activity, offering an experience of the everyday and familiar in an unfamiliar world. It also allows parents and siblings to join in with the patient in a way that they are accustomed to, giving a sense of their being able to contribute to the child's well-being. As Harvey and Hales-Tooke (1972) put it 'By occupying himself in creative activities he is, in a sense, repairing those parts of himself which he feels have been broken or damaged.'

The second aspect is the contribution of play to the child's continuing on a normal developmental trajectory. Although it is not uncommon to find that children regress when they are under stress, the 5 year old returns, for example, to 3 year old behaviour, play in hospital can help to make the experience one of growth, socially, cognitively, emotionally, and physically. An extreme example of this is found in the work carried out at Great Ormond Street several years ago with a 3 year old boy who was paralysed from the neck down. He could talk but not move anything other than his head. The ward psychologist, Jo uglas, mobilized help in all directions and was able to have a special computer-assisted environment created for him so that he could control the movements of an electric wheelchair with his mouth. Equally importantly, he could use his mouth to control a mechanical arm which allowed him to move objects on a table. As he got older and the equipment became more sophisticated he was able to paint, to build with bricks; he was even able to disobey adults by knocking his bricks over—being naughty for the first time in his life (Douglas and Ryan 1987). Less extreme but equally to be considered are the needs of long-stay children. They will, if steps are not taken, miss out on a whole range of activities that aid normal development, from travelling on a bus or a train to the experiences surrounding ordinary school. Particular attention needs to be paid to the language development of these children, whose restricted environment can lead to an impoverished vocabulary.

Related although somewhat removed from what has been said so far, is the role of the play specialist as a constant person in an ever-changing world of nurses and others who come and go on different shifts. A study in America (Crocker 1978) found that children were exposed to up to 50 or more new people in the first 24 hours of their stay in hospital. While that number may now be fewer there is still a bewildering array of new faces, which is especially critical when parents are unable to visit.

The reduction of anxiety

This is a major function of play in hospital. At the very least play offsets boredom, in itself a stress producer, while at the more productive level, it is more than just a diversion. Children who have been subjected to traumatic experiences often seem to need to repeat those experiences through play, through drawing them over and over again, through talking about them. In this way they gain some sense of coming to terms with what has happened and of gaining mastery over the otherwise overwhelming emotions they have felt.

Even if the experience of being in hospital is not sufficient to be called a trauma, there are times for many children when anxieties are aroused and play can then be a safety valve for feelings, an outlet for tensions and conflicts.

Unguided play is not, though, always likely to be helpful in reducing anxiety; the contribution of the play specialist, discussed below, is of great importance.

Speeding recovery

Play specialists are among the least well paid of all health care staff but they are not volunteers and now that so many hospitals are preoccupied with money, questions may be asked about the cost–benefit ratio of providing play in hospitals.

Apart from other reasons given in this chapter, there is one that will appeal to the accountants: play in hospital has been reported to help in speeding recovery, possibly through a reduction in the child's anxiety (Plank 1971; Billington 1972; Jolly 1975; Garot 1986).

Facilitating communication

Children often find it easier to talk when they are playing or drawing, while some communicate through their play or their artwork. One boy I knew on an oncology ward made a series of models involving coffins, while another mentioned in Chapter 5 drew a picture of a tiny sailing boat in a storm protected by two huge whales. Although there are all sorts of problems in interpreting what children produce, play specialists can work with play and drawings as a means of communication, with help from a psychologist or psychotherapist, as is discussed earlier in Chapter 5.

A number of books and a board game have been devised to facilitate communication between children and adults and they are also discussed in Chapter 5.

Preparation for hospitalization or for procedures

This is such an important topic that it has a chapter to itself (see Chapter 7).

Organized play in hospitals

What one calls people who facilitate play is a never-ending source of discussion. As Rubin (1992) notes, the psychological importance of a job title is significant and much thought has gone into the names on both sides of the Atlantic. The names given have included child care specialist, child development aide, developmental specialist, puppet lady, play lady, play specialist, patient activity therapist, recreation room teacher, recreational therapist, teacher, babysitter, and volunteer.

One of the first, if not the first, paid hospital 'play activities workers' was appointed to Johns Hopkins Hospital in America in 1944 (Wilson 1986). Although the discipline has flourished in that country ever since, it is salutory to note that even in 1990 there was some resistance there to the notion of a paid worker (Rubin 1992).

By 1960 the play activities programme in Johns Hopkins was known as Child Life, to recognize 'the more encompassing service (beyond play activity) that Child Life was offering' and workers were known as Child Life teachers, following the inclusion of school as an integral part of the programme. In 1980 the Child Life profession was formally designated and staff can now earn a nationally recognized credential as a Certified Child Life Specialist from the Child Life Certifying Commission.

In Great Britain a significant date was 1963 when the first Save the Children Fund play leader was appointed to the Brook Hospital. She was not the first in Britain, St Bartholemew's Hospital had already had one for several years, but she was the forerunner of a series of play leaders in hospitals supported by the Save the Children Fund throughout the country.

Their numbers grew apace, their worth being demonstrated in their daily work. After much debate the title play specialist was eventually chosen and the Hospital Play Staff Examination Board was set up to award qualifications; there are at present six colleges offering training and staff are now on their own pay structure, a significant step in recognizing the discipline in its own right.

The British hospital play tradition was rooted in psychoanalytic theory. Susan Harvey and David Morris, two pioneers of the movement, were experienced in that approach, but it soon broadened and is now eclectic in its theoretical orientation.

What play specialists do

To some extent it is possible to glean something from what has already been said. They work anywhere in a hospital although in many there is a designated play area on a ward or in a main hospital play centre; in larger hospitals there will be both. They are responsible for the provision of materials, they supervise volunteers, and help parents when necessary. They observe children and discuss their needs when appropriate. Above all, they guide children at play in order to help meet their emotional and developmental needs. An account of a day in the life of a play specialist is given in Digby (1992).

From the outset there has been a more or less clear definition of the play specialist's role. It has always been seen as separate from both nursing and teaching and although play specialists work with children who are distressed they do not perceive themselves as therapists. The Save the Children Fund (1989) report identifies six key elements.

1. To put play on the agenda, to have it accepted as a normal part of the routine anywhere in a hospital where children are admitted.

2. To contribute to clinical judgements of children by observing them and communicating findings to relevant colleagues.

3. To identify children and/or parents who are having difficulties in coping.

4. To introduce some normality into a child's day (a function shared with the hospital teacher).

5. To accompany children to and/or assist with particular treatments.

6. To integrate nursing staff into children's play.

This list is fine as far as it goes but it runs the risk of underestimating the positive contribution that play specialists can make to the everyday well-being of the child. Also in the Save the Children Fund (1989) report and elsewhere, for example Sylva (1987), it is clear that there is ample scope for work in the relief of anxiety, for preparation, and for working to support parents as well as children.

One of the key characteristics of play specialists is their role as members of a team. They play an important role in psychosocial meetings (see p. 99) and since the overarching construct within which they work is the notion of the whole child they see it as vital to communicate with others.

When there is no play specialist

Play is a natural part of childhood and it might be argued that children do not need someone who is paid to help them do something that they do any way. In fact young children, especially young children under stress, do not always play spontaneously (Williams 1972) and when they do they may not play as productively as when professionally supervised. Cross and Swift (1990) observed 12 young children's play and emotional state during a week, when there was a play specialist and teachers were on duty and at weekends when they were absent. Major differences were found.

Quality standards

In Britain the National Health Service has moved towards a system in which health care is seen as a form of trade: hospitals and other providers have to sell their wares in an open market. Part of the selling process is the setting of standards in certain areas and play provision has not been excluded. In the most recent survey of play provision in Britain carried out by the Hospital Liaison Committee in 1985, only 37 per cent of wards admitting more than 50 children per annum had a paid play specialist. The document entitled *Quality management for children: play in hospital*, issued by the Play in Hospital Liaison Committee in 1990, with a foreword by the Minister for Health, sums up quality standards and at the same time provides a neat summary of what play can do and what play specialists are all about. Particularly useful is the check-list which can be applied to ensure that play is adequately provided. The standards listed in that document provide a good ending to this chapter.

1. Play should be a separate service, organized by a qualified hospital play specialist.

2. Play specialists should be full members of the health care team.

3. Play specialists should be involved in advising on making the environment in all parts of the hospital more friendly for children and adolescents.

4. Play specialists should be involved in training hospital staff about the needs of children and adolescents in hospital.

5. Play services should link in with child development centres and community services.

6. All hospitals should have a staff ratio of not less than one play specialist to 10 child in-patients, depending on an assessment of needs.

7. Play staff should be paid on salary grades appropriate to their training and skills.

8. A senior play specialist should be appointed to coordinate services throughout the hospital.

9. Play services should be separately managed and accountable to general management.

10. All hospitals should have a clear policy and guidelines on the involvement of volunteers and students working with children.

References

Billington, G.F. (1972). Play program reduces children's anxiety, speeds recoveries. *Modern Hospital*, **118**, 90–2.

Crocker, E. (1978). Play programs in pediatric settings. In *Psychosocial aspects of paediatric care*, (ed. E. Gellert). Grune and Stratton, New York.

Cross, C.A. and Swift, P.G.F. (1990). Observation and measurements of play activities in a paediatric ward. *Maternal and Child Health*, **15**, 354–61.

Department of Health and Social Services (1976) *Health services development: play in children's hospitals*. Health Circular HC(76)5.

Digby, M. (1992). A day in the life. *Cascade*, **3**, 4–5.

Douglas, J. and Ryan, M. (1987). A preschool severely disabled boy and his powered wheelchair: a case study. *Child: Care, Health and Development*, **13**, 303–9.

Erikson, E. (1963). *Childhood and society*, (revised edn). Hogarth Press, London.

Freud, A. (1936). *Writings of Anna Freud vol II*, (revised edn). International Universities Press, New York.

Garot, P.A. (1986). Therapeutic play: work of both children and nurses. *Journal of Pediatric Nursing*, **1**, 111–16.

Garvey, C. (1977). *Play*. Fontana, London.

Groos, K. (1989). *The play of animals*. D. Appleton, New York.

Groos, K. (1901). *The play of man*. D. Appleton, New York.

Harvey, S. and Hales-Tooke, A. (ed.) (1972). *Play in hospital*. Faber & Faber, London.

Herron, R.E. and Sutton-Smith, B. (1971). *Child's play*. Wiley, New York.

Huizinga, J. (1955) *Homo ludens*. Beacon Press, Boston.

Jolly, H. (1975). How play in hospital helps children's recovery. *The Times*, **16 June**.

Jolly, J. (1981). *The other side of paediatrics*. Macmillan, London.

Klein, M. (1929). Personification in the play of children. *International Journal of Psychoanalysis*, **10**, 193–204.

National Children's Bureau (1992). *A charter for children's play*. National Voluntary Council for Children's Play, London.

Organisation Mondiale pour l'Education préscolaire (1966). *Play in hospital*. Report by the Organisation Mondiale pour l'Education Préscolaire.

Piaget, J. (1951). *Play, dreams and imitation in childhood*. Routledge, London.

Plank, E. (1971). *Working with children in hospitals*, (2nd edn). Year Book Medical Publishers Inc., Chicago.

Rubin, S. (1992). What's in a name? Child Life and the play lady legacy. *Children's Health Care*, **21**, 4–13.

Save the Children Fund (1989). *Hospital: a deprived environment for children? The case for hospital play schemes*. Save the Children Fund, London.

Spencer, H. (1898). *The principles of psychology*. D. Appleton, New York.

Sylva, K. (1987). Address to the National Association of Hospital Play Staff, London.

Weller, B.F. (1980). *Helping sick children play*. Baillière Tindall, London.

Williams, N. (1972). Observation of six children and how they spent one hour 11 am to 12 noon in hospital. In *Play in hospital*, (ed. S. Harvey and A. Hales-Tooke A.). Faber & Faber, London.

Wilson, J. (1986). School as a part of a child life program. In *Child life: an overview*. Association for the Care of Children's Health, Washington, DC.

7

Preparation

Introduction

The idea is simple: there is still much in hospitals that is unfamiliar, worrying, and threatening and the more one can be prepared for an event, in order to offset the fear of the unknown, the better one copes. The Platt Report (Ministry of Health 1959) was unequivocal: 'The risk that any child will be disturbed by hospital admission can be reduced by suitable preparation of both parents and children.'

Patients who have been well prepared are reported to be less anxious, require less medication, exhibit fewer maladaptive behaviours, and cope more effectively with medical procedures. They have fewer complications and do better during convalescence (Moran 1971; Azarnoff 1976; Melamed and Ridley-Johnson 1988; Peterson and Mori 1988; Yap 1988; and for a discussion on adults see Mathews and Ridgeway (1984)). Benefits have also been reported for the parents of children (Peterson and Shigetome 1981) and, a much less-often reported finding, for hospital staff (Mumford *et al.* 1982). There is also some evidence that preparation can be cost effective. R.P. Pinto and J.G. Hollandsworth (unpublished) demonstrated that patients going through a filmed modelling preparation programme stayed fewer days in hospital and used fewer medical resources than those who had not received the programme.

So we hope that the days when children were told that they were going to a party when in fact they were going to hospital, when they were told that they were going for an X-ray when in fact they were going to have a leg amputated, are long passed. We hope.

Nevertheless, it is not all plain sailing. The age and developmental status of children, their previous hospital experience, and their parents' emotional state are likely to determine the effectiveness of preparation. We need to ask questions to decide which preparation, for which procedure, for which children, will be valuable. The research addressing itself to these finer issues is discussed below.

We should also consider the possibility that knowledge in itself is not necessarily advantageous to children. Allen *et al.* (1983) showed that adolescents with a thorough understanding of their diabetes were more anxious than those who had only a superficial knowledge. In a follow-up study of survivors of Hodgkin's disease, Wasserman *et al.* (1987) found that those who were younger when diagnosed said that their lack of awareness helped them get through the experience. This was, of course, retrospective thinking and must be seen as such. Underlined is the need to consider individual children.

Preparation for hospitalization

When the admission is planned

The task begins with the knowledge that a child is likely to be admitted. Many hospitals now have some kind of *Welcome to hospital* booklet, often one for parents and another for children. That produced by Tadworth Court in Surrey is a good example: it includes a picture of the main building, information on getting there, a description of the accommodation, a list of what patients should bring with them, who the staff are, what they do and what they wear, a typical day's timetable, data on telephone numbers, and much more.

A number of general books for children have been published, many of them with a sick animal as a central character. Altschuler (1974) argued that a good one will stimulate questions as well as giving information and will also reassure that some anxiety is normal. Such books should also balance the positive and the negative aspects of the experience.

Southampton University Hospital set up a Saturday Morning Club in 1987 to help prepare parents and children, having previously already ascertained in a survey that parents felt that information giving was the crucial factor in contributing to their overall satisfaction with the care their children received. A study compared those who had attended with those who had not and found that the opportunity to learn about the admission was appreciated. However, it was noted that the club was, overall, poorly attended; reasons for not coming that were given included the cost of bus fares, the feeling that children did not need preparation, dislike of hospitals, and work commitments (Glasper *et al.* 1992).

Even if no previous preparation has been possible, children can receive some information as soon as they arrive. A major study in this context was conducted by Azarnoff *et al.* (1976) in California when 128 children aged between 4 and 11 years were seen on admission, prior to any intervention, and then assigned randomly to three groups in order to test the value of a guided tour of the hospital and of booklets introducing children to the hospital. The conclusion was that the interventions were potentially more helpful for boys who had had previous hospital admissions, where the reasons for the admission were not understood by the parents, and where only one parent was consistently involved with the child in the experience. There was a suggestion that parents need more information and that programmes to prepare children should discriminate on the grounds of age and socio-economic background, on prior experience, and understanding of the clientele. Tours appeared to be more effective than booklets for some families and were certainly better than nothing but it could not be said that they were better than booklets.

Pre-admission home visits

A certain amount has been written about the value of children being able to visit their hospital before they are admitted but rather less attention has been paid to the admittedly more time-consuming practice of a member of the ward team visiting children at home preadmission, so that when they first go onto the ward there is a familiar face to greet them. Research in this area suggests that it can be of great value (Ferguson 1979; Harris 1979).

When the admission is unplanned: anticipating hospitalization

The majority of young children in hospital are admitted as an emergency. In an American study, Poster (1983) quoting a 1978 survey, reported that approximately 86 per cent of admissions under the age of 5 years were on an emergency basis. So not only may the child arrive at the hospital unprepared, the hospital may be unprepared as well.

Helping children to anticipate going into hospital is not, however, impossible. There have been a number of attempts in America. Abbot *et al.* (1970) reported on a project in which 239 pre-school children were visited in their play group by nurses who introduced them to hospitals. Seventy-eight of the children were subsequently admitted and were found to be more settled than other patients of the same age who had not had the preparation. Pomarico *et al.* (1979) used a slide show, a hospital tour, and question and answer sessions for groups of children including some from scouts and primary schools. In Britain in the 1970s the National Association for the Welfare of Children in Hospital devised a series of pictorial games and action cards featuring various hospital procedures and situations, designed for children aged 5–7 years. Evaluations showed that colour photographs were the preferred form of illustration, that the games were effective in improving children's knowledge of hospitals, and that they were effective in reducing children's anxiety concerning an impending blood test, making them more cooperative during the procedure (National Association of the Welfare of Children in Hospital 1980; Rodin 1983).

Harley (1980) wrote up her experiences of talking to toddlers in play groups and nursery schools. She tried to include parents in the session and loaned classes some finger puppets of people in hospital plus some relevant story books. She started by asking children about their experiences of being ill at home and then moved to what would happen if they were very ill indeed. This was followed by slides of an ambulance and then some discussion of normal events in hospital, followed by some slides on play.

Eiser and Hanson (1989) set up a play hospital in a small rural primary school. Five and 8 year olds were studied and seemed to have benefited in terms of information about hospitals acquired and in the development of non-fearful attitudes towards hospitals as such.

But even these programmes may have pitfalls. As recently as 1986 a quarter of the wards admitting children to hospital in Britain also admitted adults; approximately one-third of children in hospital in Britain and up to 65 per cent in the rest of Europe are in adult wards. It could be counter-productive to prepare children for their going to a lovely hospital where there are play specialists and friendly nurses who know all about children if they are to end up in the corner of an adult ward where play never happens. The answer is probably to give general preparation rather than to be too specific, especially in making promises.

Medical staff in regular contact with children and families are often in the best position to prepare in a general way. General practitioners' surgeries are usually full of literature and a booklet on children in hospital could easily be included. Health visitors are also able to do much in this area.

Preparation for specific procedures

The principles are similar: one should try as far as possible to identify the key areas that are likely to cause distress and to prepare children and parents for them in as much detail as seems reasonable for each child.

Preparation for the painful and the unpleasant

Much of what happens to children in hospital is nasty, brutish, and long. They may lose their hair, may have a hole cut in their throat, wake up from an anaesthetic feeling far more unwell than when they went to theatre, and, above all, they may have injections. Pain is discussed in Chapter 9; here it needs only to be said that even when there is to be a really unpleasant event, it is better to be honest, for if there is evasion or a lie, the child's trust will be lost. It always helps to explain how long the pain or discomfort will last.

Preparation of all senses

Children are likely to experience changes from their normal routine in what they see, hear, touch, and smell and should be prepared in all areas.

Modelling

Encouraging children to watch a film of a child undergoing treatment and coping is one of the techniques most often quoted in the research literature. The most frequently cited study to demonstrate the value of this approach is that of Melamed and Siegel (1975) who made a 7 minute film entitled *Ethan Has an Operation*. Ethan was a real boy who had a hernia repair and in their study Melamed and Siegel (1975) found that 4–12 year olds who had seen it were less fearful and showed lower behavioural distress than controls.

Puppets have also been tried, with some success (Schulz *et al.* 1981), leading Peterson and Mori (1988) to conclude that whatever the form, film, video, or puppet, a model is an effective vehicle for preparation of children.

It is not, however, clear, what aspect of techniques such as this is crucial. Perhaps there is a desensitizing effect, perhaps the children watching learn a new set of responses from watching a peer. Perhaps the children's parents become more relaxed once they have seen another child coming through unscathed (Pinto and Hollandsworth 1984). Perhaps there is an additive effect: Peterson and Shigetomi (1981) used coping techniques such as relaxation, distraction, and self-instruction built into a preparation programme, with and without filmed modelling and concluded that a combination of the two was the optimal approach.

Play

Playing through the experience in anticipation is common on paediatric wards. It is now not unusual to go onto a surgical ward and see a child operating on a doll or removing stitches. Sometimes the whole procedure can be played, sometimes only certain parts. Once again, one has to be careful about the message given. At Great Ormond Street we have Hickman Teddy, a bear who has a Hickman catheter inserted. It was a good idea and has helped many children, but it took a while to realize that some who were prepared in this way thought that they were going to return from the insertion not only with a Hickman but also covered in fine brown hair!

The bandaging of a doll to indicate what kind of bandaging the child is likely to have, an extension of which is actually to bandage the child, is another play way to prepare. This is of great importance when children will recover from an operation to find themselves restricted. There are, for example, children who undergo cranio-facial surgery who come round from the anaesthetic with their mouths wired up so they cannot speak, bandaged in such a way that they cannot see, with mobility in only one hand. It passes one's imagination to try to envisage how a child who had not been carefully prepared would feel.

Photographs and booklets

Photograph albums are of value for procedures where there is a clear sequence of events, the insertion of a gastrostomy, for example. Children, with parental permission, are usually happy to volunteer to be subjects for this exercise and several albums can be devised with captions varying according to the developmental level of the child.

Valerie Binnie, a psychologist at Sheffield Children's Hospital, has written a booklet for children and parents to cover leg-lengthening operations. She pulls no punches, making it clear that there may be periods of boredom for everyone, that children will become dependent on their parents in a way that they used to be when much younger, that they will be in a wheelchair, and that there is some pain involved but that this will pass.

Talking

It is easy to get lost in a welter of videos, photographs, and dolls and to forget that sometimes the simplest approach is the best and one of the simplest is talking. It is essential to use the child's vocabulary: if the family refer to a tumour as such that is fine but if they call it a lump then this is the preferred term.

Other factors to be considered

Age

One of the hardest tasks I have encountered was trying to prepare a 2 year old for an arm amputation. (The play specialist and I managed this with the use of a doll whose arm came off.)

It is easy to say that the younger the children, the less likely they will be to understand the procedures and, therefore, they need no preparation. Certainly they present a problem: they are less skilled at asking questions, they recall less information, are more likely than older children to have misconceptions about the cause of their illness (see Chapter 4), and have fewer self-initiated coping strategies. All this adds up to the need to focus preparation at least as much on the pre-school group as on older children. There is much to be done to develop and evaluate techniques for the pre-school child.

Gender

There seems to be no evidence of a gender-based difference in children's responses to hospitalization or treatment (Peterson and Mori 1988).

Previous medical experience

There is some indication that the preparation of children who have previous experience of hospitalization, in general and surgery, in particular, may have to be approached differently from that of naive patients. Melamed *et al.* (1983) concluded that modelling films may be contraindicated for younger, experienced children, perhaps because of the body of misconceptions and fears that have been built up. On the other hand, my clinical experience of children who are veterans is that they can often take their in-patient admission in their stride, especially if they go repeatedly to the same ward with the same staff.

Timing

A relatively little researched area is the timing of preparation. I have sometimes asked children when they like to be told that something is going to happen and the general rule of thumb is the younger the children the less time there should be between telling them and the event taking place. This must be kept within reason, of course; I am not advocating that one prepares a young child about to have an amputation only an hour or so before. There is some experimental support for this view of age and timing from Melamed *et al.* (1976).

The implication of what has been said about timing is that all information is given at one moment. In fact, it is often better to spread it over a few days, even a few weeks, giving details just before the event when one is reasonably sure that they will be correct.

The preparation of parents

Arthur Koestler was a toddler when he was taken to have a tonsillectomy. He wrote later, 'Half senseless with fear, I craned my neck to look into my parents' faces and when I saw that they, too, were frightened, the bottom fell out of my world' (Koestler 1952).

Most published examples of preparation have focused more or less exclusively on children, yet there is something to be said for joint work. The booklet on leg lengthening mentioned above has been written expressly for both. Parental reactions to hospitals and to illness can be powerful influences on children's responses (Roskies *et al.* 1978) and it can be argued that one of the key factors in explaining the success of preparation programmes has been the incidental inclusion of parents.

Encouraging questions

Whatever method of preparation is used, it will be of limited value if there is no opportunity for children to ask questions and opportunity includes a ward atmosphere which allows this to be done comfortably. One 6 year old girl seemed preoccupied for days. Finally she came out with a question to her father, 'After my treatment is over, will I be the same person?'

Explaining why

This has been left to the end not because it is the least important but because it is, perhaps, the most important. It is not enough to explain what is going to happen; this must be accompanied, in most cases, with some explanation why. The point is illustrated in the true story of a boy, the son of two doctors, who went into hospital for an undescended testicle operation. The operation took place in the hospital where his father worked so there were no problems about pre-admission visits. The boy knew the anaesthetist socially and everyone went to great pains to explain exactly what would be done, when, and how. His parents were with him on the day of the operation.

When he returned home he was clearly distressed, to everyone's dismay. It was only later that he was able to tell his parents that what had upset him was the fact that no one had told him why he was having the operation that the penny dropped.

A preparation check-list

Does *everyone concerned* know what is to happen, how it will be done, when it will be done, why it will be done, and, how everyone will feel afterwards?

See also Chapter 15 on surgery.

References

Abbott, N.C., Hansen, P., and Lewis, K. (1970). Dress rehearsal for the hospital. *American Journal of Nursing*, **11**, 2360–2.

Allen, D.A., Tennem, H., McGrade, B.J., Affleck, G., and Raatzen, S. (1983). Parent and child perceptions of the management of juvenile diabetes. *Journal of Pediatric Psychology*, **8**, 129–41.

Altschuler, A. (1974) *Books that help children deal with a hospital experience*. US Department of Health, Education and Welfare, Washington DC.

Azarnoff, P. (1976). The care of children in hospitals: an overview. *Journal of Pediatric Psychology*, **1**, 5–6.

Eiser, C. and Hanson, L. (1989). Preparing children for hospital: a school based intervention. *The Professional Nurse*, 4, 297–300.

Ferguson, B.F. (1979). Preparing young children for hospitalization: a comparison of two methods. *Pediatrics*, 64, 656–64.

Glasper, A., Venn, C., and Roberts, A. (1992) Preparing for hospital. *Cascade*, 6, 3–4.

Harley, B. (1980). Let's play hospitals. *National Association for the Welfare of Children in Hospital NEWS No 5.*

Harris, P. (1979). Children, their parents and hospital. Unpublished PhD thesis. University of Nottingham.

Koestler, A. (1952) *Arrow in the blue*. Hutchinson, London.

Mathews, A. and Ridgeway, V. (1984). Psychological preparation for surgery. In *Health care and human behaviour*, (ed. A. Steptoe and A. Mathews). Academic Press, London.

Melamed, B.G. and Ridley-Johnson, R. (1988). Psychological preparation of families for hospitalization. *Developmental and Behavioural Pediatrics*, 9, 96–102.

Melamed, B.G. and Siegel, L.J. (1975). Reduction of anxiety in children facing hospitalization and surgery by use of filmed modeling. *Journal of Consulting and Clinical Psychology*, 43, 511–21.

Melamed, B.G., Meyer, R., Gee, C., and Soule, L. (1976). The influence of time and type of preparation on children's adjustment to hospitalization. *Journal of Pediatric Psychology*, 1, 31–7.

Melamed, B.G., Dearborn, M., and Hermecz, D.A. (1983). Necessary considerations for surgery preparation: age and previous experience. *Psychosomatic Medicine*, 45, 517–25.

Ministry of Health (1959). *The welfare of children in hospital*. HMSO, London.

Moran P. (1971). Unpublished PhD thesis quoted by Janis, I. *Stress and frustration*. Harcourt Brace, New York.

Mumford, E., Schlesinger, H.S., and Glass, G.V. (1982). The effects of psychological intervention on recovery from surgery and heart attacks. An analysis of the literature. *American Journal of Health*, 72, 141–51.

National Association for the Welfare of Children in Hospital (1980). *London National Association for the Welfare of Children in Hospital NEWS No 5.*

Peterson, L. and Mori, L. (1988). Preparation for hospitalization. In *Handbook of pediatric psychology*, (ed. D.K. Routh). The Guilford Press, New York.

Peterson, L. and Shigetome, C. (1981). The use of coping techniques to minimise anxiety in hospitalized children. *Behavior Therapy*, 15, 197–203.

Pinto, R.P. and Hollandsworth, J.G. (1984a). An evaluation of psychological preparation of pediatric surgery using videotape models. Unpublished manuscript quoted in Eiser, C. (1990) *Chronic childhood disease*, Cambridge University Press.

Preparation

Peterson L., Mori L. (1988) Preparation for Hospitalization. In *Handbook pediatric psychology*, (ed D.K. Routh), The Guilford Press, New York.

Pinto, R.P. and Hollandsworth, J.G. (1984) *Preparing parents of pediatric surgical patients using a videotape model*. Paper presented at the meeting of the Society of Behavioral Medicine, Philadelphia.

Pomarico, C., Marsh, K., and Doubrava, P. (1979). Hospital orientation for children. *AORN Journal*, 29, 864–70.

Poster, E.C. (1983). Stress immunization: techniques to help children cope with hospitalization. *Maternal Child Nursing Journal*, 12, 119–34.

Rodin, J. (1983) *Will this hurt?* Royal College of Nursing, London.

Roskies, E., Mongeon, M., and Gagnon-Lefebvre, B. (1978). Increasing maternal participation in the hospitalization of young children. *Medical Care*, 16, 765–77.

Schulz, J.B., Rashke, D., Dedrick, C., and Thompson, M. (1981). The effects of a pre-operational puppet show on anxiety levels of hospitalized children. *Journal of the Association for the Care of Children's Health*, 9, 118–20.

Wasserman, A.L., Thompson, E., Wilimas, J.A., and Fairclough, D.L. (1987). The psychological status of survivors of childhood/adolescent Hodgkin's disease. *American Journal of Diseases of Children*, 141, 626–31.

Yap, J.N. (1988). A critical review of paediatric preparation procedures: process, outcomes and future directions. *Journal of Applied Developmental Psychology*, 9, 349–87.

8

Emotional factors

Introduction: the nature of stress

It is easy to argue that children and their families are, often but not always, under great stress in hospital. It is harder to grapple with the meaning of the word, for it is overused, frequently misunderstood. 'The single most remarkable historical fact concerning the term ... is its persistent, widespread use in biology and medicine in spite of almost chaotic disagreement over its definition' (Mason 1975).

The word is derived from the Latin 'stringere' meaning to draw tight. It was used in the seventeenth century to describe hardship and affliction. In the eighteenth century it came to mean pressure, strain, or strong effort. Early in the twentieth century came the idea of stress causing disease. What, though, does the word actually mean in the context of this book? The literature is at first sight confused, leading one author to conclude that it is particularly difficult to work out what experience or psychological state 'stress' is supposed to be referring to. Is it, he wonders, a generic term for all negative feelings or just another word for threat or anxiety? Does it lead to negative feelings or is it a consequence? (Duckworth 1985).

A psychological definition is offered by Varni and Wallander (1988): 'The occurrence of problematic situations requiring a solution or some decision-making process for appropriate action.' This, however, seems to miss the essential point which is that stress is something which can cause distress. A neater definition is that it is the result of a mismatch between perceived demands and perceived resources. Put another way, one can say that what causes suffering is not the amount of pressure that is put on a person, it is the realization that one cannot come up with the goods, that one does not have the capacity to respond to what is seen to be demanded.

The crucial factor, then, is individual perceptions. If we go into any ward where children suffer from similar conditions we will find a myriad of responses to the demands made by the illness. Faced with a blood test, one child will grimace stoically, another will scream but keep still, while a third will kick and struggle. The idea of individual differences in this context throws into relief the need to allow that a trivial episode in the eyes of an adult can be of immense gravity for a child. We can also use this standpoint when considering parental stress and, of course, staff stress (see Chapter 19).

Anxiety

Anxiety is another 'buzz' word that requires elaboration. One way of looking at this is to see it as a feeling that arises when one cannot predict what is going to happen. The fear of the unknown is one of those cliché phrases that contain an essential truth: the more unknown our future is the more likely we are to be anxious about it. As one father put it, 'I could cope if I knew my daughter was going to get better; I could cope if I knew she would die; it's not knowing that's so hard.' An example common to everyone is the experience of going to a new school or place of work. Even the most insensitive people are liable to a twinge of anxiety on their first day—a twinge which disappears as the setting becomes more familiar. For some people hospital is a breeding ground for anxiety, from the moment they enter to find inadequate signposting to the time they leave, having not been prepared for what was going to be done and having not understood a word of the doctor's explanations.

Emotional adjustment

When discussing the extent and nature of what, for want of a better term, can be called emotional adjustment among children and their families we find that the picture is confused. It is confused partly because we are dealing with two sets of phenomena: one is those directly to do with being in hospital, the other is related to children being so ill that they have to be in hospital in the first place. This chapter takes each in turn.

Emotional adjustment and hospitalization

Going into hospital does not appear to be the hazard it once was, for the anxiety about the extreme emotional effects of hospitalization, evident in the 1940s and 1950s, has now passed. Shannon *et al.* (1984) in a birth cohort study of 1265 children in New Zealand, followed up at the age of 6 years, found a slight increase in behaviour problems associated with the length of stay in hospital but they disappeared when socio-economic and life event variables were taken into account. The report concluded, 'There is little evidence to suggest that in a modern pediatric setting admission to hospital has any significant effect on the child's subsequent behavioural pattern.' Similar findings were reported in the United States by McClowry and McLeod (1990) when they found no significant changes in pre- and post-admission behaviour in 50 children aged between 8 and 12 years.

On the other hand, hospitals are, to quote one young patient, 'places where they hurt you'. No matter how friendly the staff, there are inevitable sources of distress, many of which cannot be overcome. It is to be expected, then, that some children will, some of the time, become disturbed by their experiences. To illustrate this, Cross (1990) studied 50 children in a British hospital, taking the ability to settle back into previous behaviour patterns as a criterion for successful adaptation. She found, in a heterogeneous sample of medical and surgical patients, with ages ranging from 2 to 7 years and stays varying from 1 day to a little more than 1 week, that 54 per cent showed some problems in settling. Neither the presence of the mother, nor the length of admission or whether the admission was the child's first had any effect on outcome. But perhaps most interesting was that most of the difficulties reported passed within 6 weeks, thus providing support for the New Zealand study quoted above.

An example of the effects of rare and demanding treatment is found in a study by Pot-Mees (1989) of children with leukaemia undergoing bone marrow transplantation, involving a long stay in isolation, which indicated that 35 per cent of them had significant behaviour problems 1 year after discharge. In this study the effects of a serious illness were controlled for, so one cannot look just at the leukaemia as a cause of the distress.

The fact that children can be upset by being in hospital even if their mothers are present throughout and that in extreme cases this distress can last for a year or more can be explained in terms of discontinuity theory. The notion, put forward by Margaret Stacey and her colleagues, is that the greater the discontinuity between home and hospital the greater will be the distress. It would be hard to imagine a greater discontinuity than that experienced in bone marrow transplantation. This, then, goes beyond the ideas of Bowlby and others on maternal separation, indeed, one of the books from this group is entitled *Beyond separation* (Hall and Stacey 1979).

Much effort has been made in recent years to make hospitals more homely: Basildon Hospital has children taken to theatre on a Thomas the Tank Engine trolley, white coats are a rarity, and children are encouraged to bring in photographs, pillow cases, videos, and toys to remind themselves of home. But even when massive steps are taken to offset the differences there will still be some strange aspects; it is easy for people who work in hospitals to underestimate how frightening they can be to others. There will still also be pain and discomfort.

The challenges and problems presented by chronically sick children

The extent of the problem

The literature is confusing: the Ontario Child Health Study (Cadman *et al.* 1987) concluded that children who are ill are twice as likely to have psychological disorders as healthy children, yet one can read in a recently published American text, 'Most children with chronic illness do not manifest psychological disturbance or maladjustment.' Later on the same page: '...this population is at increased risk for mental health and adjustment problems' (Garrison and McQuiston 1989). In another, British text, one finds 'It is clear that some children with chronic disease show an increased risk of maladjustment but many children show no measurable deficits.' Four pages later in the same book comes: 'Several large-scale epidemiological surveys indicate that children with chronic disease are at a greater risk of maladjustment than healthy peers' (Eiser 1990*a*).

There are six main reasons to explain these apparent contradictions.

One is that there is no general agreement on what is meant by the term 'adjustment'. As Eiser (1990*a*) has pointed out, adjustment, adaptation, coping, stress, competence, and dysfunction are used interchangeably. This is far more than just a question of playing with words. Some children are described as having a psychiatric disorder, that is, they behave abnormally, but it is highly questionable to use criteria for psychopathology which have been developed from physically healthy populations when considering children who are sick. The child or parent who uses denial, asserting firmly that all will be well come what may, is using a defence mechanism but this could be seen as healthy—necessary to avoid a complete emotional breakdown.

A second cause of confusion is found in the way that adjustment is often measured. Most studies use rating scales and parents or some other adult fill in check-lists to rate behaviour and to come to a conclusion on the child's emotional state. But it is possible that these scales are insufficiently sensitive to pick up the stress felt by children. The boy in the corner of the classroom, the one with the disfigured face, may score zero on a behaviour rating scale, may be described as quiet, giving no trouble. What no-one but he knows is the strain of coping with the stares, the teasing, the looks of horror that his appearance evokes. He may not be 'maladjusted' but he is not without his psychological problems.

A third reason is related to the second: people do not always agree in their opinions on a child's behaviour; even parents can vary quite markedly (Eiser *et al.* 1992).

A fourth reason lies in the wide range of samples used to collect data. Some studies use large populations, for example all the children born in a certain week or living in a certain area. An often-quoted example of this is the Isle of Wight study (Rutter *et al.* 1970). Others draw on smaller samples from clinics or hospitals. They can and do provide valuable information but may be biased, for example by focusing too much on one social class or ethnic group.

Fifth is the failure always to realize the importance of taking the age of the child into account when determining adjustment. It has been shown, for example, that the special needs of children with diabetes vary with age (Rovet *et al.* 1987).

Finally, just as there is no consensus on the definition of adjustment, so there is no universally accepted theory underpinning research in this area.

With all that in mind, we can try, cautiously, to come to some very general statements.

A recent review (Eiser 1990*b*) concludes that 'The weight of scientific evidence continues to point to the increased vulnerability, in terms of emotional and behavioural development, of children with a chronic disease.' She quotes a study of 3294 children in Canada aged 4–16 years in whom the incidence of chronic disease was 14 per cent, including 3.7 per cent of children who also suffered from physical disability of some kind. Children with chronic disease and physical disability were at more than three times the risk of psychiatric disorder and at 'considerable' risk for social maladjustment compared with healthy children. Those with chronic disease but no physical disability were at a two-fold increased risk of psychiatric disorder but were not significantly different from healthy children in social adjustment.

Along with this can go the finding that children whose medical conditions include involvement of the central nervous system have an undoubtedly increased risk of behaviour disorder. Breslau (1985) for example, looked at children with cystic fibrosis, cerebral palsy, multiple physical handicaps, and healthy controls. Using the Psychiatric Screening Inventory in which mothers report on children, she found that those with cystic fibrosis had significantly less psychopathology than other groups with brain involvement. The risk of psychiatric impairment was, incidentally, directly related to the degree of intellectual functioning.

We can say with some certainty that there is little if any evidence that an early episode of chronic illness *per se* has an effect on the person's emotional state at later ages. Thus, in one longitudinal study, Orr *et al.* (1984) concluded that 'The simple presence of a chronic medical problem 8 years earlier did not seem to place the child at increased risk for subsequent psychosocial problems.' On the other hand, anxieties about the possible return of a disease have been noted, at least for former cancer patients (Koocher and O'Malley 1981). Once again, we are back at the recurring theme: these survivors of cancer may not be 'disturbed' in that they are able to function perfectly well but illness-related emotional problems exist for them.

The nature of the disturbance

Despite attempts to identify them, consistent personality traits associated with particular conditions seem not to exist; we cannot talk of the diabetic personality or the asthmatic personality or the cancer personality. We can, however, point to certain behavioural trends in some cases: children with a facial disfigurement tend to be a little more withdrawn than others, children with well-controlled diabetes seem to show more than the average amount of depression (Close *et al.* 1986; Fonagy *et al.* 1987).

There are differences of opinion on how justified one is in lumping together all diseases when discussing psychological factors. Should we not see the problems presented by asthma as essentially different from those of leukaemia or cerebral palsy?

To some extent there *are* broad differences. Children whose condition is life threatening are not identical with those who cannot walk.

The emotional sequelae of a condition like autism, when there is so little interaction with the child, are not to be compared to those of eczema.

On the other hand, there is a school of thought which stresses the similarities that hold at least across chronic conditions. This so-called non-categorical approach (Varni and Wallander 1988) sees families of all children with a chronic condition confronted by a series of similar stresses: hospitalization, expense, the need to make special arrangements for siblings, for transport, for school, and so on.

Eiser (1993) argues that what is important is not the label attached to the disease but the extent to which it disrupts the family's ability to maintain everyday activities.

Gender

There is little if any evidence to indicate significant gender differences in response to hospitalization (Sylva and Stein 1990).

Previous experience

Research findings are equivocal, some finding no effects of previous admissions, others showing that children who have been in hospital before show more distress on subsequent admissions (Sylva and Stein 1990).

Age

A number of studies have shown that younger children show more distress than those who are older (Vernon 1967; Katz *et al.* 1980; Jay *et al.* 1983) but there is always the possibility that older children are more adept at hiding their feelings.

Adaptation and the severity of the disease

Psychology has been described as no more than common sense dressed up in statistics. This is an unfair description for common sense is extremely fallible: after all, common sense tells us that the world is flat. Common sense would also tell us that a child with a major physical condition is more likely to be disturbed than one whose problem is relatively light. A careful examination of children shows that while this is sometimes the case, as, for example, in asthma (Maclean *et al.* 1992) this is not necessarily so. Perrin *et al.* (1989) report a curvilinear relationship, whereby children with moderate asthma were better adjusted than those with either mild or severe forms of the illness. Wallander *et al.* (1989*a*, *b*) failed to establish any link between maternal and child adjustment and severity of disease in cerebral palsy and spina bifida. Indeed, there is some evidence to suggest that just the opposite is true: children with the most serious physical problems often seem better able to cope than those whose problems are mild (McAnarney *et al.* 1974). Drotar and Bush (1985) reviewed the topic and concluded, 'Disease severity based on objective physical criteria may not be as important as personal perceptions of illness in mediating adjustment.' As was noted at the beginning of this chapter, stress is very much related to the person's individual perception of demands and resources.

Cognitive functioning and school attainment

Of the many anxieties expressed by children in hospital those related to missing school are amongst the easiest to understand and, to some extent at least, to deal with. We have here an example of the need to consider developmental factors: frequent school absences can play havoc with examination programmes and it is sometimes necessary for a child to repeat a year. Although there is little systematic evidence on this topic, anecdotal accounts suggest that younger children do not necessarily fall badly behind in reading and can catch up quite quickly in mathematics.

More subtle effects, more long lasting also, are those impairments associated with certain medical conditions. Some are directly to do with the disease. Children with cerebral palsy, for example, score right across the range from the very low to the very high on intelligence tests but the average for such children is lower than the national average for the unimpaired. Any disease which may involve the brain leads to greater vulnerability as far as schoolwork is concerned. We are, to risk repetition, looking at averages here: there are many highly intelligent children with, for example, cerebral palsy but their existence does not invalidate the argument.

Sometimes the learning difficulty can be caused by the treatment rather than the illness itself. It has been suggested that some of the medication prescribed for asthma lead to deficits in visuo-spatial abilities and memory (Creer 1987). There is ample support for the idea that the interventions used for children with leukaemia have resulted in cognitive impairment, especially in memory, in a significant number of children (Fletcher and Copeland 1988).

The family and the sick child

One of the more facile remarks in the literature on childhood disability is that which asserts that a handicapped child means a handicapped family. By extension one could argue that a sick child means, if not a sick family, at least one which is dysfunctional. There is some support at least for the idea that having a sick child increases the likelihood of parental disturbance. Hughes and Lieberman (1990) found that one-third of the parents of children with cancer, even including those in remission, had such anxiety and depression that they needed professional help. A similar figure has been quoted for mothers of children with diabetes (Davis 1993).

One myth can be dispelled: having a sick child undoubtedly puts a huge burden on parents but there is no good evidence whatsoever that parents of chronically sick children are more likely to divorce than others.

There is always the need to avoid an overdependent relationship building up. This can occur very easily when a child requires a great deal of help in everyday matters. For example, there is a skin condition, fortunately rare, known as epidermolysis bullosa. Children suffering from extreme forms of this illness have to have dressings changed every day, a process that can take up to 2 hours a time. They find it painful to walk because their feet blister and sometimes have restricted use of their hands. It is in cases like this that one sometimes finds a child who has become overdependent on his or her mother, with the equally unfortunate result that other members of the family feel, correctly, that they are being neglected.

There is also a tendency towards hypervigilance in families of sick children: one sneeze and mother is in a tizzy.

The family and hospitals

When a child goes into hospital the family will be thrown off balance. No matter how trivial the cause, any in-patient admission and many out-patient appointments bring anxiety and uncertainty in their train. In recent years there has been an emphasis on seeing families in terms of a system: if one member changes in some way the others will all adapt in some way themselves, for good or ill. A number of character-istics of the healthy family have been considered in this context all of which have relevance for the child in hospital.

First, just realizing that their system will be affected can be a help. One teenage girl in a family where this was not acknowledged burst out one day, 'I'm fed up with having to make allowances for my sister.' The problems of siblings are discussed further below.

If the child is seriously ill there will be a stream of enquiries from friends and family, a strain in itself. (It helps at times like this to set up an arrangement by which a close friend or relative acts as a messenger to others. Parents relay information to this person who then takes on the task of passing it on to others in the neighbourhood.)

Parents who stay in with a child often complain of boredom and fatigue: 'It's more tiring sitting here than going to work.' More dis-tressing is the often-voiced sense of having been deskilled as parents as they have had to hand over the care of their child to others. The move in some hospitals to involve parents in medical care is a partial response to these complaints.

As before, when we were looking at children themselves, it is virtually impossible to disentangle the specific problems brought about by the strains of being in hospital from the results of the illness itself. An added complication is that financial resources may have an effect as well.

One of the problems in coming to conclusions from the literature is that so much emphasis has, so far, been put on mothers, the role of fathers having been somewhat neglected. Another is that researchers have often been preoccupied with seeking out ways in which families have failed to cope rather than looking at what they have done that is functional.

Family income, social class, and coping

The literature on economic factors is clear and not surprising in its conclusions: the more money you have the easier it is to cope. One study looked at parental incomes and maternal educational levels in 153 families with children aged 4–16 years suffering from six different conditions. When mothers' reports of children's adjustment and family relationships were analysed it was found that both financial and psy-chological variables were related to the child's adjustment, in particu-lar in social spheres. Similar findings were reported by Anderson *et al.* (1983) when it was noted that asthma was associated with the financial state of the family.

Some caution is needed in the interpretation of studies on costs of treatment from America since the expense of medical treatment is so high there. In Britain, although treatment in National Health Service hospitals is free, fares for visiting, time lost from work, and the purchase of extra presents can put a huge strain on a tight budget. One mother in a children's hospital parent support group said one day that she and her husband were reaching the end of their tether and had decided to have a long weekend in the Bahamas. Another mother, a single parent, commented ruefully that the nearest she ever got to a holiday was watching the advertisements on television.

There is yet a further complicating factor, rather harder to study, related not just to simple income but to social class. As was discussed above in the section on discontinuity theory, hospitals can be intimidating places, despite the efforts to make them more friendly. The medical profession has a reputation for arrogance, despite the efforts of many present practitioners to overcome barriers. The more articulate, confident parents are likely to find themselves better able to deal with the extra pressures that they are exposed to.

Before we go into a spiral of stereotypes it must be said that there is no evidence of a one to one relationship between income and/or social class and coping. As so often happens, we are talking here of averages and trends rather than individuals.

Siblings

Always mentioned, often ignored, siblings of sick children suffer themselves in silence. This is an overstatement but it has more than a grain of truth. Some surveys of siblings of sick children suggest that they have lower self-concepts, can be socially isolated, and resentful of parents' involvement with the sick child (Eiser 1990*b*). On the other hand, one study of 48 siblings of boys with pervasive developmental delay, diabetes, and healthy controls found no support for the idea that the siblings of the ill children were uniformly at greater risk of psychosocial impairment than siblings of those who were healthy. The author did conclude that siblings of the same sex as the ill child have more problems than those of the opposite sex but since only sick boys were included this must be treated with caution (Ferarri 1984). Unfortunately although many professionals working in hospitals agree that siblings are a vulnerable group there is rarely the opportunity to do very much about them.

Too much should not be made of all this. It is easy to be dazzled by data about life-threatening conditions and chronic handicap: in fact most children are in hospital for only a short period for an acute rather than a chronic problem. On the other hand, there are some characteristics of hospital which affect all children, no matter why or for how long they are in. There is stress; everyone has to cope.

Coping in hospital

We talk of people coping when we see them managing to survive, even to function well, in the face of adversity. The notion of stress and coping is central to an understanding of the psychology of the sick child for we are not, in general, faced with children and families who are mentally ill, rather we find people who have perfectly normal reactions to abnormal situations. If you have severe asthma, kidney disease, cystic fibrosis, or any other serious condition it is hardly surprising that there will be times when you and your family are sad, anxious, or angry.

A definition of stress was given at the beginning of this chapter, if we say we are to try to help people cope with abnormal stress we should also try to understand what we mean by the term coping.

The process of coping has been defined, following the definitions given above, as 'efforts ... to manage ... environmental and internal demands, and conflicts among them, which tax or exceed a person's resources' (Lazarus and Launier 1978).

Surprisingly little has been written about how children cope with stress. Rutter (1981) suggests that more intelligent children may cope better because they have more mature conceptions of the situation. One of the few studies directly on the topic is that by Wertlieb *et al.* (1987). They asked school-aged children how they dealt with stressful experiences and concluded that girls actively sought support more than boys, with greater use of all strategies with increasing age. Several studies have been carried out on how children cope with pain. Reviewed in Chapter 9 they suggest that left to their own devices younger children in particular have few strategies. Much has also been done under the banner of preparation, so much that it is discussed separately in Chapter 7.

When thinking about how well children and their families cope with hospitalization, it helps to try to analyse just what it is they have to cope with. One approach to this is to list the tasks facing them as Moos and Tsu (1977) have done.

1. Dealing with pain and incapacitation.

2. Dealing with the hospital environment and developing relationships with the hospital staff.

3. Preserving emotional balance by managing feelings of anxiety, resentment, and isolation.

4. Preserving a positive self-image.

5. Preserving relationships with family and friends.

6. Preparing for an uncertain future.

Not all of these are relevant for all children, of course. Someone coming in for tonsillectomy, for example, *should*, in normal circumstances, not have doubts about the procedure and its consequences; pain is not an inevitable concomitant of hospitalization and a short admission will not, for most children, bring a noticeable break in relationships with family and friends. Once again we have to bear developmental factors in mind: a separation of a few days from one's mother is one thing at the age of 13 years; it is very different at the age of 13 months. However, the list of tasks is a useful starting point. Issues of pain and the preparation for an uncertain future are discussed in later chapters, the task of dealing with the hospital environment is one to be taken up now.

Coping styles

A recent review of research on the coping styles children use when faced with stressful medical procedures has concluded that they can be divided into the active, information-seeking approach or the avoidant, information-denying style (Peterson 1989). It seems likely that the former are less anxious, more cooperative, and show higher tolerance for pain than the latter. Whether the differences in anxiety and the rest are simply to do with style or whether the style chosen is a marker for an underlying difference between the groups of children is not easy to answer. The review does, however, support the need for parent involvement and preparation of children so that information may be available. (See Chapter 7 on preparation.)

Communication

The more open communication can be between family members and between family and staff, the better the psychological outcome (Koocher and O'Malley 1981). The more closed the communication system the more chance there is of children having fantasies about the unknown, with an increase in anxiety. An extreme example of this came with a family who told the sibling of a sick child nothing at all about the illness beyond the fact that his brother was in hospital. They did not tell the truth even when the child died, keeping quiet on the subject for 2 years.

Open communication should be matched with a regard for each family member's privacy; we all need to get away sometimes. Open communication with staff is equally important, as is communication between staff. Here there can be some modelling; when families know that the staff are all aware of what is going on because they have a good communication system they will be that much more confident in communicating themselves. How often, though, does a member of staff wonder aloud what has been said by others or, worse, give messages which contradict those of others? (See also Chapter 5 for a further discussion on communication.)

Creating a more normal environment

The realization of the need to reduce discontinuity has led many hospitals to try to become more user friendly, as was mentioned above. Pre-admission visits, information leaflets, a relaxed atmosphere between the staff, parents, and patients all add up to making hospital more home-like.

Hospital schools have a big part to play in normalizing children's lives as well. A well-equipped, well-staffed schoolroom and teachers who can visit the wards of those children who are unable to get to the class, can offer far more therapeutically than may be apparent at first.

More and more children's units or hospitals now have a local radio. It may be part of a network, like Radio Lollipop, or it may be independent. Either way there should be an opportunity for patients and siblings to join in the making and the broadcasting of programmes designed specially for them. I have known a number of children who now look forward to admission because they can contribute to the radio activities.

Then there are animals in hospital who may replace much-loved pets. Flopsy was an adored rabbit who lived in a hospital playroom, petted, stroked, cared for by hundreds of children. Some animal lovers provide a service to hospitals, visiting them with guinea-pigs or whatever, so that children may relate to them on a regular basis.

On at least one occasion a rabbit did far more for a child's mental state than the ward psychologist. Janey was in hospital miles from home. She was very sick indeed and was missing her sister and her dog. All sorts of approaches were tried to help her lift her depression but none was as successful as the rabbit brought in by the Wood Green Animal Shelters. Janey found she could not only help to look after the rabbit, she had someone she felt confident in talking to as well. (See the end of the chapter for the main address of the shelters.)

Other ways of helping

All this may not be enough. What can be done for those children who are severely upset or depressed? Several approaches have been tried. One is to give them permission to be depressed or anxious. The nurse who says, 'Come on, cheer up, long face' is not being very helpful. The one who indicates that she understands that the child is low and that this mood is reasonable in the circumstances, will be in a position to help to take steps to overcome the depression, anxiety, or whatever.

One of the best ways to help people is to make demands on them. A number of children have been helped enormously by their having been asked to do something around the ward or the hospital. One boy, with enough physical disabilities to make anyone morose, is like a lark whenever he is admitted because he has been befriended by the porters. He helps them to such an extent that he has been given an ID badge, bearing his photograph and the title 'honorary porter'.

Children separated for a long period from their families often enjoy keeping a log book of what they have done and what has happened to them. This is part diary and part scrapbook and is described in Chapter 5.

When children are alone and sometimes parents simply cannot or will not come in or even visit regularly, it may be possible to find a volunteer to act as a surrogate parent, what has been called a ward granny (Jolly 1981). With careful selection and supervision this can work well, especially for the vulnerable very young child who is not developmentally able to make friends with peers. It can be a disaster, as with the volunteer who is unreliable or the one who cannot cope with the distress evidenced by the child or the one who becomes so emotionally attached to the child that he or she needs help to let the patient go at the end of the admission.

A multidisciplinary approach

In the last 10–20 years there has been a growth in the multidisciplinary approach to the psychosocial problems of children and their families. This involves ward-based staff working alongside others: chaplains, psychiatrists, psychologists, and social workers, not only in a fire-fighting, crisis management mode but in a more rounded way, looking at issues concerning the staff as well as the patients (Black *et al.* 1990).

Some hospitals have a weekly psychosocial meeting, similar to a ward round but focusing on the emotional and social needs of children and their families. At their best these provide an opportunity for planning the admission of patients who are known to be a problem, for the discussion of present patients and their management, and for catching up on past patients. They can also act as a forum for the discussion of tensions or stress on the ward. An example of this came on one occasion when a parent had complained about a junior doctor and the nursing staff felt that the complaint was justified. They were concerned lest nothing was done about it. After a long discussion it was agreed that the sister would tell the doctor and the consultant of the staff's concerns.

Predicting adjustment

One way of summarizing much of what has been said in this chapter is to look at an often-quoted model to predict adjustment in mothers of sick and handicapped children which has been put forward by Wallander *et al.* (1989*c*). They follow the currently commonly adopted view that we are looking at multifactorial causes of adjustment and look to two sets of factors: one set related to risk and the other to resistance.

Under the heading risk come those factors to do with the following.

1. The disease or disability: medical factors to do with the severity of the condition, whether it is visible or not, whether it involves the brain and/or cognitive functioning, etc.

2. Functional independence.

3. Psychosocial stressors which include major life events, what are described as 'daily hassles', and handicap-related problems.

Under resistance come three groups.

1. Intrapersonal factors: temperament, competence, problem-solving, ability etc.

2. Social ecological factors: the family environment, the extent of social support available, family members' adaptation, and economic resources.

3. Stress processing, the ability to appraise what is happening and to take coping action.

Together these lead to greater or lesser adaptation evidenced by the parent's mental and physical health and social functioning. Although this work was done in the context of disability in general, it can be applied to families of children in hospital as well.

Observing adjustment

Since the late 1970s there has been an interest in measuring the distress shown by children in hospital and over the years techniques have become increasingly sophisticated, although remaining relatively simple to administer. A useful short review of what has been done plus a detailed description of the Observational Scale of Behavioural Distress (Elliott *et al.* 1987) is given in an article by Sylva (1992).

Hospital as a positive step

Reams have been written on how awful hospitals were and quite a lot is published on the problems that still arise, yet for some children a spell as an in-patient can be a rewarding experience. Work on the resilience of children (Rutter 1987) has argued that with care, children can use hospitalization as a 'steeling' experience, to help them withstand subsequent stresses the better. The key here is that children have to be helped to cope with the experience. We are a long way from the 'What is wrong with emotional upset?' question mentioned in Chapter 2.

A rather less happy benefit of hospital comes when it is a more pleasant place to be than home. I have had a handful of children referred to me because they were refusing to leave.

Sometimes the reason is clear, as in the case of the teenage girl with a facial disfigurement whose parents were, to say the least, unsympathetic. On the plastic surgery ward she was regarded as normal.

Sometimes it is related to the amount of attention children receive in hospital and do not receive at home. One boy, whose younger brother had died, was neglected at home, it seeming that his parents had given up on him. He said quite openly that he liked attention and went to considerable lengths to gain it.

Sometimes it is related to unwanted attention at home: a child who is being physically or emotionally abused by a family member will feel safe in hospital.

Sometimes it relates to the order and care given in hospital which contrasts with chaos at home.

Whatever the reason, we should not underestimate the power for good that the hospital experience can bring.

When parents are a problem

It is easy to talk of the child who presents staff with problems; it is not uncommon for criticisms to be levelled at hospital staff or management for being insensitive or uncaring; but it is relatively rare to find published comments on the difficult parent, other than those with a clearly defined problem such as Munchausen syndrome by proxy, which is discussed in Chapter 12. Yet parents are not perfect and there should be an acknowledgement that this is so.

In an unpublished account of one summer on a paediatric ward, the psychologist to that ward has described how having more than one difficult mother at one time caused immense distress to the staff, especially the nursing staff.

The behaviours that were noted were as follows.

1. Manipulativeness: playing off one member of staff against another, talking in a derogatory way to staff about their colleagues.

2. Disturbances in mood, especially mood swings: 'One minute she was all smiles and the next she was screaming.'

3. Rough or neglectful treatment of their children, while showing affection whenever a doctor came round.

4. Whipping up complaints from the other mothers.

5. Obscene language.

6. Lying.

7. Interfering with the care of other children.

The result of having more than one mother showing some or all of these behaviours was the creation of an extremely unpleasant atmosphere on the ward. Fortunately, there was a regular psychosocial meeting at which feelings could be explored and shared and fortunately there was an opportunity to seek help from a psychiatrist who explained some of the pathology involved. But not all wards have psychologists and psychiatrists on hand, not all by any means have regular psychosocial meetings. For them the difficult parent may be the last straw in the creation of intolerable stress. (See also Chapter 12 on Munchausen syndrome by proxy.)

References

Anderson, H.R., Bailey, P.A., Cooper, J.A., Palmer J.S., and West, S. (1983). Morbidity and school absence caused by asthma and wheezing illness. *Archives of Disease in Childhood*, **58**, 777–84.

Black, D., McFadyen, A., and Broster, G. (1990). Development of a psychiatric liaison service. *Archives of Diseases in Childhood*, **65**, 1373–5.

Brain, D.J. and Maclay, I. (1968). Controlled study of mothers and children in hospital. *British Medical Journal*, **1**, 278–80.

Breslau, N. (1985). Psychiatric disorder in children with physical disabilities. *Journal of the American Academy of Child Psychiatry*, **24**, 87–94.

Cadman, D., Boyle, M., Szatmari, P., and Offord, D. (1987). Chronic illness, disability and mental and social well being: findings of the Ontario Child Health Study. *Pediatrics*, **79**, 805–13.

Creer, T.L. (1987). Psychological and neurophysiological aspects of childhood asthma. In *Childhood asthma: pathophysiology and treatment*, (ed. D.G. Tinkelman, C.J. Falliens, and C.K. Napitz). Marcel Dekker, New York.

Cross, C. (1990). Home from hospital. *Nursery World*, **15**, 22–3.

Davis, H. (1993). *Counselling parents of children with chronic illness or disability*. British Psychological Society, Leicester.

Drotar, D. and Bush, M. (1985) Mental health issues and services. In *Issues in the care of children with chronic illness*. (ed. N. Hobbs and J. Perrin). Jossey-Bass, London.

Duckworth, D.H. (1985). Is the 'organizational stress' construct a red herring? A reply to Glowinkowski and Cooper. *Bulletin of the British Psychological Society*, **38**, 401–4.

Eiser, C. (1990*a*). *Chronic childhood disease.* The University Press, Cambridge.

Eiser, C. (1990*b*). Psychological effects of chronic disease. *Journal of Child Psychology and Psychiatry,* **31,** 85–98.

Eiser, C. (1993). *Growing up with a chronic disease.* Jessica Kingsley, London.

Eiser, C., Flynn, M., Green, E., Havermans, T., Kirby, R., Dandeman, D., and Tooke, J.E. (1992). Coming of age with diabetes: patients' views of a clinic for under-25 year olds. *Diabetic Medicine,* **10,** 285–9.

Elliott, C.H., Jay, S.M., and Woody, P. (1987). An observation scale for measuring children's distress during medical procedures. *Journal of Pediatric Psychology,* **12,** 543–51.

Ferarri, M. (1984). Chronic illness: psychosocial effects on siblings—I. Chronically ill boys. *Journal of Child Psychology and Psychiatry,* **25,** 459–76.

Fletcher, J.M. and Copeland, D.R. (1988). Neurobehavioural effects of central nervous system prophylactic treatment of cancer in children. *Journal of Clinical and Experimental Neuropsychology,* **10,** 495–538.

Garrison, W.T. and McQuiston, S. (1989). *Chronic illness during childhood and adolescence.* Sage Publications, London.

Hall, D. and Stacey, M. (ed.) (1979). *Beyond separation: further studies of children in hospital.* Routledge & Kegan Paul, London.

Hughes, P. and Lieberman, S. (1990). Troubled parents: vulnerability and stress in childhood cancer. *British Journal of Medical Psychology,* **63,** 53–64.

Jay, S.M., Ozolins, M., and Elliott, C.H. (1983). Assessment of children's distress during painful medical procedures. *Health Psychology,* **2,** 133–47.

Jolly, J. (1981). *The other side of paediatrics.* Macmillan, London.

Katz, E.R., Kellerman, J., and Siegel, S. (1980). Behavioural distress in children with cancer undergoing medical procedures: developmental consideration. *Journal of Consulting and Clinical Psychology,* **48,** 356–65.

Koocher, G.P. and O'Malley, J.E. (ed.) (1981). *The Damocles syndrome.* McGraw-Hill, New York.

Lazarus, R.S. and Launier, R. (1978). Stress-related transactions between person and environment. In *Perspectives in international psychology,* (ed. L.A. Pervin and M.P. Lewis). Plenum, New York.

Maclean, W.E., Perrin, J.M., Gortmaker, S., and Pierre, C.B. (1992). Psychological adjustment of children with asthma: effects of illness severity and recent stressful life events. *Journal of Pediatric Psychology,* **17,** 159–72.

Mason, J.W. (1975). A historical view of the stress field. Part 1. *Journal of Human Stress,* **1,** 6–12.

McAnarney, E., Pless, J., Satterwhite, B., and Friedman, S. (1974). Psychological problems of children with chronic juvenile arthritis. *Pediatrics,* **53,** 523–8.

Mcclowry, S.G. and McLeod, S.M. (1990). The psychosocial responses of school-aged children to hospitalization. *Children's Health Care*, **19**, 155–61.

Moos, R.H. and Tsu, V.D. (1977). The crisis of physical illness: an overview. In *Coping with physical illness* (ed. R.H. Moos). Plenum Press, New York.

Orr, D.P., Weller, S.C., Satterwhite, B., and Pless, I.B. (1984). Psychosocial implications of chronic illness in adolescence. *The Journal of Pediatrics*, **104**, 152–7.

Perrin, J., Maclean, W.E., and Perrin, E. (1989). Parental perceptions of health status and psychologic adjustment of children with asthma. *Pediatrics*, **83**, 26–31.

Peterson, L. (1989). Coping by children undergoing stressful medical procedures: some conceptual, methodological and therapeutic issues. *Journal of Consulting and Clinical Psychology*, **57**, 380–7.

Pot-Mees, C. (1989). *The psychological effects of bone marrow transplant in children*. Eburon, Delft.

Rovet, J., Ehrlich, R., and Hoppe, M. (1987). Behaviour problems in children with diabetes as a function of sex and age of onset of disease. *Journal of Child Psychology and Psychiatry*, **28**, 477–91.

Rutter, M. (1981). Stress, coping and development: some issues and some questions. *Journal of Child Psychology and Psychiatry*, **22**, 323–56.

Rutter, M. (1987). Psychosocial resilience and protective mechanisms. *American Journal of Orthopsychiatry*, **57**, 316–31.

Rutter, M., Tizard, J., and Whitmore, K. (1970). *Education, health and behaviour*. Longman, London.

Shannon, F.T., Fergusson, D.M., and Dimond, M.E. (1984). Early hospital admissions and subsequent behaviour problems in six year olds. *Archives of Disease in Childhood*, **59**, 815–19.

Sylva, K. (1992). Observational measures for assessing distress during medical treatment. *Newsletter of the Association for Child Psychology and Psychiatry*, **14**, 24–7.

Sylva, K. and Stein, A. (1990). The effects of hospitalisation on young children. *Newsletter of the Association for Child Psychology and Psychiatry*, **12**, 3–8.

Varni, J.W. and Wallander, J.L. (1988). Pediatric chronic disabilities: Hemophilia and spina bifida as examples. In *Handbook of pediatric psychology*, (ed. D. Routh). Guilford Press, New York.

Wallander, J.L., Varni, J.W., Babani, L., Banis, H.T., DeHeen, C.B., and Wilcox, K.T. (1989*a*). Disease severity and psychosocial adaptation in children with cerebral palsy. *Journal of Pediatric Psychology*, **14**, 23–42.

Wallander, J.L., Feldman, W.S., and Varni, J.W. (1989*b*). Disease severity and psychosocial adaptation in children with spina bifida. *Journal of Pediatric Psychology*, **14**, 89–102.

Wallander, J.L., Varni, J.W., Babani, L., Banis, H.T., DeHeen, C.B., Wilcox, K.T., and Banis, H.T. (1989*c*). The social environment and the adaptation

Emotional factors

of the mothers of physically handicapped children. *Journal of Pediatr. Psychology*, **14**, 371–8.

Wertlieb, D., Wiegel, C., and Feldstein, M. (1987). Measuring children's coping. *American Journal of Orthopsychiatry*, **57**, 548–60.

The main address of the Wood Green Animal Shelters is Heydon, Nr Royston, Hertfordshire SG8 8PN. Telephone: 01763 838328.

9

Pain

Introduction

Top of the list of psychological problems identified by ward sisters in a survey carried out at Great Ormond Street Hospital a few years ago was the children's fear of injections. While they provide the majority of painful experiences injections are not alone: migraine, post-operative pain, and pain associated with cancer are just three of the many other sources encountered in hospital.

Pain in babies

There has been little short of a revolution in thinking about pain in babies since the mid-1980s. Until then it was commonly believed that babies probably do not feel pain since the necessary neural pathways are not developed. This meant that, horrifying though it now seems, neonates were at times operated on with an anaesthetic to only paralyse them. It is now known that although the messages may take longer to reach the brain in a young infant, they certainly do get through (Fitzgerald 1994).

Current thinking indicates that we should give sufficient analgesia not only to remove pain during an operation but also to reduce the massive shock reaction that is experienced when little or no analgesia is used (Wolf 1994). If this is done, babies suffer fewer post-operative problems; critically ill babies have an increased survival rate (Anand 1990).

Children's understanding of pain

Before trying to begin to help children cope with pain it helps to start by trying to establish their perception of its cause, its nature, and its duration. Most published work is based on Piagetian theory. An example is work carried out in Ireland by Gaffney and Dunne (1986, 1987). Six hundred and eighty children aged 5–14 years took part, a wide social class range being represented. One finding was that children could undoubtedly remember their experiences vividly, dispelling the myth that pain is less critical for them than for adults. What is more, even the youngest had grasped the concept that pain is universal. When children were asked to define what pain is they showed a shift from thinking in concrete terms to the more abstract. Young children were limited to the physical, immediate, aversive nature of pain while the older ones expressed notions of pain being a mental as well as physical phenomenon, having psychosocial effects, and sometimes possessing survival value.

Fourty-four per cent said that people bring pain upon themselves, a striking proportion, especially common being a response related to having eaten either too much or the wrong food. Other studies have reported school-aged children as perceiving intrusive procedures and surgery as threats and hostile acts (Peters 1978). It is not quite certain, however, that the children in the Gaffney and Dunne (1986, 1987) study really thought that pain was a punishment, they might have been seeking rather a simple cause and effect model. Psychological causes and effects increased with age; an example of an effect given by an older child being, 'it makes you feel weak and sometimes bad tempered with others'.

The unpleasant nature of pain was noted by all Gaffney and Dunne's (1986, 1987) age groups but older children added something: feelings of helplessness, anxiety about the duration of pain, and about its significance. These are particularly interesting findings for those working in hospitals.

The younger children's attempts to gain relief from their pain reflected their thinking: they used methods that were both concrete and passive, medication and the help of parents and medical staff being examples, while the older ones described more active approaches like rubbing the afflicted part.

Significantly, very few children of any age seemed to have developed self-initiated coping strategies.

Not all studies have supported the idea that children's thinking proceeds in neat stages. Ross and Ross (1984) studied 994 children aged between 5 and 12 years in Northern California, assigning them to categories of experience of hospitalization and of pain rather than age. Their conclusion was that knowledge and understanding for most of the sample were at a low developmental level, with no clearly defined age trends.

Ross and Ross (1984) agreed with other studies in some ways. They noted a low use of coping strategies and a 'disquietingly high' frequency of maladaptive pain usage. ('Whenever I don't want to go to swimming practice, I grab my stomach and moan and make a face like eating a lemon and I say, "Gee, mom, I *hope* I don't have to miss *swimming*"' (an 8 year old girl).)

Ross and Ross (1984) also looked at the notion of immanent justice, the idea that pain (or any other discomfort) is caused by some recent misdeed. There was only one example of a child perceiving pain as punishment: 'I forgot to take the trash out on Friday and that's why I broke my leg.'

Leaving aside the arguments of developmental psychology about stage theory one can come to some conclusions on the implications for clinical practice of academic work.

One is the possibility that children *may* construe painful procedures as some form of punishment; this may not be found often but it should be taken into account. It underlines the need not only to warn children that a certain procedure is likely to be painful but also to explain why it is being undertaken.

Linked with this is the need to explore the child's idea about the possible duration of pain and its wider meaning. The possibility of pain messages being helpful in indicating that something is wrong can be explained to quite young children.

Perhaps the most important practical finding from the studies mentioned is the evidence that, left to themselves, children rarely seem to develop coping strategies. This is where the bulk of help can be directed.

Assessment

Pain, anxiety, and distress

One of the knottiest of problems in this field is deciding what it is that we are assessing when we talk of measuring pain: are we or the children rating pain or the anxiety associated with it? It might be better to talk of distress in order to encompass both.

The context of the pain

Context in this sense means the apparent causes or surrounding factors thought to be related to the expressed pain. Sometimes it seems that there is a straightforward, immediate cause of discomfort, a finger prick is a good example. On the other hand, a headache could have any number of causes. From this initial information one can decide what further investigations may be required: in some cases a medical examination may be needed, in others a family interview, a school report, an educational assessment, an individual interview with the child, or any combination of these. Even if the cause seems simple enough to us, we should, nevertheless, still make sure that the child fully understands what is happening and why.

The intensity of pain

Observational scales are probably the most reliable techniques for assessing the outward expression of pain and anxiety. Trained observers watch children and note certain specified behaviours. The Procedure Behavior Rating Scale (PBRS) developed by Katz *et al.* (1980), the Expressive Pain Interaction Coding System (EPICS) devised by Russell (1984), and the CHEOPS (McGrath *et al.* 1985) are examples.

However, what children feel may not relate to how they behave. Jay *et al.* (1984) found in one study of 4–6 year olds that while behavioural measures of distress were correlated with physiological measures they were not so associated with children's self-reports. Adolescents in particular may try to put on a brave face, hiding their distress. It is, therefore, worth considering more than one measure.

Self-reports

Face scales are popular: a row of simply drawn faces, ranging from one with a big smile to one with tears and a downturned mouth, is shown to the child who marks the one most representative of the pain or discomfort experienced.

Many children like to use a visual analogue scale, a 'pain thermometer' being an example. This is a simple pictures of a thermometer, with one end marked zero indicating no pain, while a 10 at the other end of the line shows the position of the most pain possible. The child draws a cross along the line according to how much pain is experienced at each procedure. Even simpler is to give a pain score, from 0 out of 10 to 10 out of 10, the explanation being given that 10 is the worst possible sensation.

Questionnaires

A number of questionnaires include measures of emotional and situational variables, for example, the Children's Comprehensive Pain Questionnaire (McGrath 1987) and the Varni–Thompson Paediatric Pain Questionnaire (J.W. Varni and K.L. Thompson, unpublished) which has child and adolescent versions. These include drawings of the human body so that children can colour in that part of the body where the pain is, using their own choice of colours to indicate intensity.

The Pain Assessment Tool for Children (PATCh)— a combination of measures

The authors of this pain assessment tool, Quereshi and Buckingham (1994) point out that the wide age range of children on most wards means that up to three pain scales may have to be employed since none is suitable for the whole age range. Their version combines faces, outline body shapes, simple descriptions, a visual analogue scale, and observations and is illustrated in Fig. 9.1. It is not intended that this tool be used in its entirety for all children; it does offer a validated technique with components which can be selectively used for all children, alone or combined, from birth onwards.

Helping children cope

Painful procedures

Preparation
Anyone who has worked in a hospital paediatric department for more than 12 seconds knows how important preparation is. To say, 'This won't hurt' when it is well known that what will follow will be painful is a recipe for disaster.

Preparation for invasive medical procedures is now a well-established way of helping both children and their parents and should always be built in as part of the treatment. A number of studies have shown preparation to reduce both pre- and post-surgical distress and pain (Melamed and Siegel 1975).

Central to all preparation is information giving: both to give some idea of the noises, smells, and physical sensations that a child is likely to experience, for example, cleaning the area of skin to be injected is

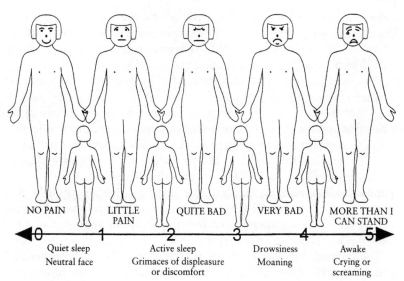

NO PAIN   LITTLE PAIN   QUITE BAD   VERY BAD   MORE THAN I CAN STAND

0   1   2   3   4   5

| Quiet sleep | Active sleep | Drowsiness | Awake |
| Neutral face | Grimaces of displeasure or discomfort | Moaning | Crying or screaming |

Fig. 9.1 The Pain Assessment Tool for Children (PATCH).

likely to feel cold and also to describe the actual steps of the procedure: what is going to be done and when (Johnson *et al.* 1975).

Anderson and Masur (1983) have found a combination of sensory and procedural preparation to be most effective.

Information

Part of the routine questioning that should take place when painful procedures are the topic of work is the extent to which the child really understands what is being done. Adults often go to some lengths to explain how important a procedure is, but this may not be enough, for there can still be a gap: not just why this finger prick/injection or whatever, is so important but also what is really being done. To say, 'Well, the doctor is taking your blood to examine it', may be enough for some children but not for others. The latter group can benefit from a detailed discussion of mechanics, including, if possible, a visit to the laboratory to see just what happens to the blood.

Alongside information giving is the opportunity to rehearse the forthcoming procedure through drawing, colouring, reading stories, puppet shows (Cassell 1965), doll play using medical equipment (Dimock 1960), and modelling films. Allowing children to play out the procedure using a favourite toy or story gives clues to what they

have understood (or misunderstood) about the forthcoming procedures, encourages expression of emotion, and facilitates the advance
of 'work of worrying', such that self-assurance mechanisms can be
called on during the procedure itself (Janis 1958).

The process of preparation is most effective when it is two way, that
is when children themselves contribute by asking questions, by indicating what more or less they want to know, and so on. Encouraging
questions and the expression of underlying misconceptions and fears is
just as important as conveying procedural and sensory information.

It is very easy for adults to fail to realize the depths of children's
misunderstanding. One child who knew that her blood count was low
panicked every time she had a finger prick because she thought that
blood being taken would mean the count going even lower. The fear
of awakening during surgery and feeling pain is not unknown as is the
fear of not waking up after surgery.

The interval between notifying the child and the actual procedure
can be crucial. Even children of 5 years can often say how much
warning they would like, be it minutes or hours. In an ideal world we
would stick to the decided time, so the child is given a sense of control
and predictability over the schedule but this is not always possible in a
busy ward with a harassed house officer.

Interventions

Most of the intervention procedures reported in the literature are for
injections, blood tests, bone marrow aspirations, lumbar punctures,
cardiac catheterizations, burn treatments, and dental care. Although
there is no great body of research literature on procedures such as
endoscopies, angiograms, and other types of catheterization, the interventions described below are equally applicable.

Whatever the technique selected, it is vital to convey to the child (and
family) that the child is learning a new skill which will enable him or
her to have a greater sense of control. The parent, play specialist, psychologist, nurse, or whoever is teaching the technique does something
with rather than *to* children, helping them to help themselves.

Permission to make a noise

It is silly to pretend that a needle does not hurt and not always helpful
to go on about how important it is to be brave. One of the simplest
coping messages is to say, 'Shout as much as you like—but keep still.'
I know one doctor who shouts along with the child, somewhat to
everyone else's surprise.

Participation

Some children have such high levels of anxiety that when faced with a painful procedure they can think about nothing else; all the carefully planned and practised coping mechanisms go out of the window. Encouraging them to participate can sometimes help. They might be allowed to choose the site of the injection/venepuncture, swab the site, wash saline through in the case of a Hickman line, then select and stick a plaster. This sounds good in theory but participation can easily slip into prevarication: 'I want it in my left arm, no, my right ... wait a minute, I want my mum here... no, I want her on the other side of the bed ... where's my dad? I want him here, too ...' Half an hour later the needle is still not in.

Distraction

Distraction is an age-old method of helping at times of acute distress and has been shown to be very successful indeed (Kuttner *et al.* 1988). However, it involves far more than a matter of simply saying, 'cooee, look over there'. The key is to make the activity interactive; the more the children join in the more their interest and enthusiasm will be held.

Infants can be distracted and soothed with stroking, with nursery rhymes or songs, while they suck a dummy; for older babies, watching an adult blow soap bubbles from a wand and then patting or catching them, action rhymes such as 'round and round the garden' and 'pat-a-cake' can all be used. Toddlers can blow bubbles themselves while the adult encourages them to blow away the scary or painful feeling along with the bubbles (Kuttner 1991). Pop-up books are often a great source of distraction, as are, for some children, computer games.

As soon as children can count a whole range of strategies opens up. They can look through a book to count the number of times a certain object appears, they can count in twos as high as they can, they can count backwards or backwards in threes. They can be invited to spot the deliberate mistake in counting that an adult makes.

All children like stories; some young children enjoy a variant of their favourite story with a surprise or unexpected event added to maintain attention and interest. Others, of course, hate any change in their favourite. Coping skills can be enhanced by the introduction of the child's favourite character into a story; this character then undergoes the same medical procedure as the child. It sometimes helps if the favourite character is frightened, just a little and manages to overcome the fears while acknowledging that the procedure was unpleasant, thus providing the child with a role model. Suggestions for mastery over painful sensations can be included in the story. A favourite addition is the magic glove: the child meets a hero who tells all about a special, invisible 'magic glove'. When the glove is put on sensations of pain or discomfort are greatly reduced. It adds to the effect if the putting on of a glove is mimed during the telling of the story.

Desensitization

This is the classical approach to fears, in children as well as adults (Barrios, *et al.* 1981). The basic principles are well known: that one allows the child to relax and to encounter whatever is feared in a graded, step by step way, the child deciding on the pace of the treatment, so that the feared object becomes associated with a comfortable emotional state, with the child in control, rather than one of terror.

Children who are frightened of needles can start with a picture of a needle, they look at it, handle it, perhaps even colour it in. Next comes the opportunity to play with a toy medical kit. We can learn a lot about children's feelings from observations of how they jab the needle into a doll or an orange.

Next a real needle can be introduced and then the needle is gradually brought closer to the skin, eventually allowing the point to touch the skin. This sequence should be discussed first with the child in detail, with the child establishing the hierarchy of events. As a technique it is often helpful but can be quite time-consuming.

Modelling

The idea behind this approach is that if children can see someone else coping, they will be able to manage better themselves, especially if the person coping is another child. Sometimes children watch other children but more frequently a film is used, for example in preparation for surgery (Melamed and Siegel 1980). A choice has to be made between two types of model. Mastery models display no anxiety, they cope smoothly and effortlessly, putting out their arm for a needle, sitting in a composed manner throughout the session. Coping models on the other hand exhibit initial anxiety but then go on to manage successfully. Not surprisingly, Meichenbaum (1971) found that children identify more easily with coping models.

A review of the behavioural treatment of children's fears by Graziano *et al.* (1979) suggests that a combination of modelling and desensitization is particularly effective for blood tests. A combination of filmed modelling and coping techniques has been found more effective than either modelling or coping techniques alone in the preparation of children for surgery (Peterson and Shigetomi 1981).

Cognitive–behavioural interventions
The heart of cognitive work is the notion that there is no such thing as an event, only the perception of an event, so what one has to do is help children perceive the procedure or even the pain in a different light, a technique sometimes called 'reframing'. One boy who had to undergo lumbar punctures imagined that he was a spy who had been captured by the enemy. If he made a noise he was betraying his comrades. The pain was no less intense but much more bearable.

Cognitive–behavioural strategies are often presented as a selection of techniques from which the child can choose. The programme developed by McGrath and colleagues (Lascelles *et al.* 1989) for adolescents with migraine consists of a package of cognitive and behavioural techniques.

Cognitive–behavioural psychology is a growth industry and more reports of its use are likely to appear in coming years (Peterson and Shigetomi 1981; Jay *et al.* 1987).

Chronic pain

The interventions discussed below can be used for painful procedures to great effect but they are also useful in cases of chronic pain.

Guided imagery, relaxation, and hypnosis
Guided imagery   Some children prefer to get right away from the hospital, in their minds at least, by the fantasy of being in a favourite place or occupied with a chosen activity. When I am using this approach with children I sometimes call it 'directed daydreams'. Once again, we should always try to have a sense of cooperation with children rather than imposing our ideas of what their fantasy ought to be. We may choose a tropical beach or a mountain resort as a relaxing location for ourselves, whereas children often prefer an adventure. We have often been requested to devise stories involving falling into snake pits, being chased by a tiger or roaring dinosaur, only to be told the stories were 'OK but not scary enough'.

Hypnosis   There is no accepted definition of hypnosis. Some argue that it is no more than deep relaxation and guided imagery, while others insist that it produces an altered state of consciousness. The distinction is blurred by some authors who refer to hypnosis or guided imagery as though they were synonymous. Indeed, some argue that many of the distraction techniques described above could be called examples of hypnosis. Further confusion can be caused by the use of the term 'hypnotherapy' as distinct from hypnosis. A common distinction is to employ 'hypnotherapy' to refer to the therapeutic use of hypnosis.

However it be defined, hypnosis is frequently reported as a coping technique and its efficacy is now very well documented (Hilgard and Le Baron 1984; Kuttner 1991).

In practice, whatever words may be used to describe it, therapists who work in this area follow much the same sequence of activities. First children are made comfortable, then attention is focused and they are helped to reach a state of relaxation, often quite deep. This is followed by a guiding of the child's thoughts in a way that will help to bring relief of some kind. A frequently used image is the pain switch: children are told that they are in a special room with a set of switches that they can turn to reduce their discomfort. This is especially helpful in the case of chronic pain.

Finally, the child is gradually brought back to the present time and place, with much ego strengthening comment on how well he or she has done.

While good story-telling may involve several of the components of hypnosis, those techniques involving very deep relaxation and guided imagery are not without their dangers and should only be carried out under the supervision of trained, experienced staff.

Matching the intervention to the child

Developmental factors

Intellectual ability and emotional development are more important considerations than chronological age for it is very easy to underestimate the sophistication of some 3–4 years olds and to fail to realize that even a streetwise teenager may enjoy playing with a cuddly toy in hospital. Even blowing bubbles can be successfully used with children up to and beyond adolescence, for example when combined with guided imagery. The child is asked to visualize the colour of the pain, place it on the bubbles or on an imaginary cloud, and float it away across the room. As the pain moves off the bubble or cloud changes to the child's favourite colour.

Parental behaviour

Most children want their parents present during a procedure. In a study of 720 normal children aged 9–12 years, Ross and Ross (1984) found that 99 per cent reported that, irrespective of the pain experienced, the 'thing that helped most' was to have parents present.

There are, however, exceptions to this rule. Jay *et al.* (1987) showed a strong positive relationship between parental anxiety and child distress during bone marrow aspirations. When parents themselves are terrified of needles, blood, or hospitals or are still coming to terms with the shock and distress of a diagnosis, their emotions are often conveyed to their children and one of the earliest pieces of negotiation may be with the parent rather than the child.

When all else fails

With the best will in the world there are some children who continue to kick and scream no matter how many attempts are made to help them. One boy who fell into this category, a large teenager, dusted himself down after a struggle to take blood and said, 'There, that's better, you should just hold me down—forget all that psychological nonsense.'

He had a point about being held, although I would see this as still within the realm of psychological interventions. For some children it is kinder to tell them that we have to get on with the procedure, whether they like it or not and that we want to get it over as quickly as possible. These children should not have to wait any longer than they have to once they have arrived in the clinic or treatment room and if necessary they should be wrapped in a blanket to stop them hurting others. As long as this is done in a way that does not convey the child is being punished it is to be recommended as a last resort and, in conveying that the adults are in control of the situation, may provide a message of security to the child.

Afterwards

Rewards, stars, stickers, and trophies can effectively promote the confidence and self-esteem with which the child faces future medical procedures. But rewards should not just be for bravery; they should aim to give the message that the child's attempt to master difficult situations has been appreciated. The reward is given for trying to cope, whatever the outcome. Even if a child has great difficulty complying, a reward emphasizes that the child has endured the procedure.

A few children, as previously described, resist all attempts at preparation and distraction; for them playing out the procedure after it is all over may be a helpful means of achieving mastery. Many children spontaneously play out procedures on dolls or puppets using toys or real medical equipment. Carefully supervised needle play sessions (using real needles and syringes) are extremely popular. Many a child has been observed ferociously attacking a doll or orange with a needle, with evident satisfaction and relief.

Conclusion

The techniques described above have been shown to be effective with a great many children. The key concepts are as follows.

1. Putting children and parents in control as much as possible.

2. Using families' own resources.

3. Continuing to try even if at first one's ideas have not been as successful as one had hoped. It is when a child says, 'Perhaps I should try ...' that we know we are on to a winning streak.

References

Anand, K.J.S. (1990). Neonatal stress responses to anaesthesia and surgery. *Clinics in perinatology,* **17**, 207–14.

Anderson, K.O. and Masur, F.T., III (1983). Psychological preparation for invasive medical and dental procedures. *Journal of Behavioural Medicine*, **6**, 1–40.

Cassell, S. (1965). Effect of brief puppet-therapy upon the emotional responses of children undergoing cardiac catheterization. *Journal of Consulting Psychology*, **29**, 1–8.

Dimock, H.G. (1960). *The child in hospital: a study of his emotional and social well-being*. Davis, Philadelphia.

Fitzgerald, M. (1994) The neurobiology of fetal and neonatal pain. In *Textbook of pain* (ed. P. Wall). Churchill Livingstone, Edinburgh.

Gaffney, A. and Dunne, E.A. (1986). Developmental aspects of children's definitions of pain. *Pain*, **26**, 105–17.

Gaffney, A. and Dunne, E.A. (1987). Children's understanding of the causality of pain. *Pain*, **29**, 91–104.

Graziano, A., De Giovanni, K., and Garcia, K. (1979). Behavioural treatment of children's fears: a review. *Psychological Bulletin*, **86**, 804–30.

Harbeck, C. and Peterson, L. (1992). Elephants dancing in my head: a developmental approach to children's concepts of specific pains. *Child Development*, **63**, 138–49.

Hilgard, J.R. and Le Baron, S. (1984). *Hypnotherapy of pain in children with cancer*. Kaufmann, Los Altos, CA.

Hurley, A. and Whelan, E.G. (1988). Cognitive development and children's perception of pain. *Pediatric Nursing*, **14**, 21–4.

Janis, I.L. (1958). *Psychological stress*. Wiley, New York.

Jay, S.M., Elliott, C.H., Katz, E.R., and Siegel, S.E. (1984) *Assessment of children's distress during painful medical procedures*. Paper presented at a meeting of the Society of Behavioral Medicine, Philadelphia.

Jay, S.M., Elliott, C.H., Katz, E.R., and Siegel, S.E., (1987). Cognitive–behavioural and pharmacologic interventions for children's distress during painful medical procedures. *Journal of Consulting and Clinical Psychology*, **56**, 860–65.

Jeans, M.E. and Gordon, D. (1981). *Developmental characteristics of the concept of pain*. A paper presented at the 3rd World Congress on Pain, Edinburgh.

Johnson, J., Kirchoff, K., and Endress, M. (1975). Altering children's distress behaviour during orthopaedic case removal. *Nursing Research*, **24**, 404–10.

Katz, E.R., Kellerman, J., and Siegel, S.E. (1980) Behavioral distress in children with cancer undergoing medical procedures: developmental considerations. *Journal of Consulting Psychology*, **48**, 356–65.

Kuttner, L. (1991). Special considerations for using hypnosis with young children. In *Clinical hypnosis with children*, (ed. W.C. Wester, II and D. O'Grady). Bruner Mazel, New York.

Kuttner, L., Bowman, M., and Teasdale, J.M. (1988). Psychological treatment of distress, pain and anxiety for young children with cancer. *Journal of Developmental and Behavioral Pediatrics*, **9**, 374–81.

McGrath, P.A. (1987). The multi-dimensional assessment, management and research of pain syndromes in children. *Behavioural Research and Therapy*, **25**, 251–62.

Meichenbaum, D.H. (1971). Examination of model characteristics in reducing avoidance behaviour. *Journal of Personality and Social Psychology*, **17**, 298–307.

Melamed, B.G. and Siegel, L.G. (1975). Reduction of anxiety in children facing hospitalisation and surgery by use of filmed modelling. *Journal of Consulting and Clinical Psychology*, **43**, 511–21.

Melamed, B.G. and Siegel, L.G. (1980). *Behavioural medicine: practical applications in health care*. Springer, New York.

Peters, B.M. (1978). School aged children's beliefs about the causality of illness: a review of the literature. *American Journal of Maternal and Child Nursing*, 7, 143–54.

Peterson, L. and Shigetomi, C. (1981). The use of coping techniques to minimize anxiety in hospitalised children. *Behavior Therapy*, 12, 1–14.

Quereshi, J. and Buckingham, S. (1994). A pain assessment tool for all children. *Paediatric Nursing*, 6, 11–13.

Ross, D.M. and Ross, S.A. (1984). Childhood pain: the school-aged child's viewpoint. *Pain*, 20, 179–91.

Russell, S.W. (1984) Development of a behavioral interaction coding system for pain expression of children. Unpublished doctoral dissertation. University of Utah.

Scott, R. (1978). 'It hurts red.' A Preliminary Study of Children's Perception of Pain. *Perceptual Motor Skills*, 47, 787–91.

Wolf, A.R. (1994) Pain in babies: hard to identify but essential to diagnose and treat. *Cascade*, 13, 4–5.

Further reading

Jay, S. (1988). Invasive medical procedures. In *Handbook of pediatric psychology*, (ed. D.K. Routh). The Guilford Press, New York.

McGrath, P.J. and Unruh, A. (1987) *Pain in children and adolescents*. Elsevier, Amsterdam.

McGrath, P.J., Johnson, G., Goodman, J.T., Schillinger, J., Dunn, J., and Chapman, J. (1985). The CHEOPS: a behavioral scale to measure post operative pain in children. In *Advances in pain research and therapy*, (ed. H.L. Fields, R. Dubner, and F. Cervero). Raven Press, New York.

Olness, K. and Gardner, G.G. (1988) *Hypnosis and hypnotherapy with Children*. Grune and Stratton, Philadelphia.

10

Life-threatening conditions

Introduction

This chapter is concerned with those children whose life is threatened by their illness over a long period. It does not look directly at those who are involved in an accident or whose illness is sudden in onset, rapid in progress, although much that is discussed may be relevant.

The timetable

There is a timetable, beginning with the first stirrings of anxiety and the diagnosis. Next comes a period of mixed hope and despair when treatment may be tried and tried again. Next, for some, comes the third phase, when death approaches and, finally, comes death and mourning. The emotional needs of families varies according to what phase they are in and how they cope within it.

In the case of congenital conditions the diagnosis may come early after a child is born, in others there may be many months of anxiety, when parents believe that something is wrong but medical staff tell them they are fussing unnecessarily. Parents are full of anecdotes about the way they learned of their child's condition. Some tell of sensitive, caring hospital staff, who were able to take into account the psychological state of the family when they told of the predicted future. Others recount horror stories of brusque midwives, unfeeling doctors, who fling a label into the air and leave. Whatever the antecedents, this is an emotionally laden time, when parents appreciate sympathy but need, first of all, honest information and, if there is any treatment available, brisk reassurance about what is possible.

Children old enough to understand are no different, they benefit from being given a picture of why they are ill, what the treatment will be like, and, if possible, how long it will last. Naturally the detail of it is said will depend on the child's developmental level but some information should be given to any child with language. It helps to give a name to the illness; children are much less fazed by words like cancer than adults and they need a label, if only to be able to answer friends' questions.

As the illness progresses, families need constantly to be updated with information but they come also to appreciate emotional support from staff. This can come in formal counselling sessions from one of the psychosocial team, it can also come from other parents individually or in a group.

As death approaches there is still a need for information; 'What will she die of?', 'Will there be much pain?' This is the time that emotional support and sympathy come to the fore.

Support for families

If people are to help in times of crisis they must be trusted and perceived as genuinely caring. Many parents make little use of the help offered by staff because they have a network of family or friends at home, in their church, or in some other community. Others use hospital staff well, but in the latter case there is usually a time of getting to know each other before the support really begins. It helps if there is a message from the outset that emotional care is part of the package offered by the hospital.

Despite what has been said above about the need for briskness at first, empathy shown by professionals is appreciated. One mother, having been given bad news by a young house officer, said afterwards, 'Margaret isn't a proper doctor yet, she was in tears.' While I would never advocate professionals breaking down into uncontrollable sobs I have enough experience of working with parents to know that an expression of sorrow when it is felt does nothing but good.

Children, too, depending on their age and level of development, benefit from the knowledge that someone out there understands what they are feeling. Like their parents, they will also need someone to answer their questions, a point taken up later.

So often parents say that they feel isolated; their friends and neighbours are embarrassed because of the child's illness and do not know what to say. There is the other side of the coin: some parents do not know how to behave. As one father put it, 'I get cross when people don't ask about Hanna and I get cross when they do.'

Groups of parents sharing an experience, when everyone knows that the others are in the same boat, can be enormously supportive. A father spoke movingly to others of how he felt when he heard his daughter's diagnosis, to be met with another child's mother, who he had never met before, saying, 'Oh, I could kiss you for saying that, I thought I was the only person in the world who had that feeling.'

Other parents also understand the need to go over and over certain moments. The constant repetition of 'how I heard about my child's diagnosis' can be boring to friends (one of the reasons that some friends drop away) but not to other parents who recognize their own needs to work through the traumatic experience.

The role of the group leader is deceptively easy. An observer might say that all one does is sit there and let the parents get on with it. It is not like that. The groups I have worked in have all been unstructured in the sense that there is no formal agenda; parents can pick up on whatever they need to, but they have not been anarchic. Someone has to keep boundaries, to stop two people talking at once, to encourage gently the shy members, to stop politely one or two hogging the whole meeting, and to bring the session to a comfortable close. I have always found it valuable to be joined by a female co-worker, for so often the parents themselves need parenting and a mother and a father figure can do this more easily than one person.

Parents may, however, not feel that a group is for them; they may prefer to get to know one member of staff and relate to that person.

Individual support can take many forms. At one end of the spectrum there is the long session, an hour or so, when worries are poured out and confronted. At the other end is the 5 minute chat by the bedside about the latest soap on television, a chat which indicates that one is still around. Sometimes there are no words. One mother greeted me with, 'Come in, but I can't talk.' I sat with her, holding her hand for a quarter of an hour. Later she said how much she had valued my just being there.

Siblings

Once home from hospital the sick child remains the centre of attention, more often than not spoiled beyond belief and the well siblings may easily be left out. Because of the distance many families have to travel it is not always possible to offer very much support to them but they have as much right to information, empathy, and sympathy as anyone else. Sara Finlayson, a psychologist at Alder Hey Hospital, has developed a service for siblings of children with cancer which includes open days to visit various departments and to meet each other. Siblings can also elect to meet a staff member individually if they wish.

One warning, though: it is not a good idea to give a sibling more information than is given to the sick child, assuming that they are more or less close in age. This was done in one family and the well child became disturbed, telling his psychiatrist that the real trouble was that he could no longer hit his brother when they quarrelled because he knew and his brother did not that he was very sick. While there were probably other reasons for that child's disturbance, the inhibition from what he saw as normal behaviour exemplified much.

The postcard approach

Dora Black, a London child psychiatrist, with many years' experience of work in this field, carries a few postcards with her. From time to time she sends one to a family she has been working with, with the simple message, 'Thinking of you.' It says so much.

Communicating with children about death

In 1973 Claire Mulholland published a book of poems, written to her dead daughter. The shortest was

> Worst of all was the agony
> of not knowing
> what you knew

If we can use every means at our disposal to give children information, to communicate with them and to allow them to communicate with us at least some of this fog-like agony will be dispelled.

I know I'm going to heaven, but how will I get there? (a 6 year old).

Wouldn't it be wonderful to live to be 16? (a 13 year old).

I'm so angry, it's all been such a waste, I won't even be able to take GCSEs (a 15 year old).

These remarks and questions illustrate one of the key points in dealing with children with a life-threatening illness: the need to facilitate communication, for children may want to express fears, worries, anger; they may need also to ask questions, to explore in anticipation what is likely to happen to them and how, but they may not have the skills to open the conversation. They may, on the other hand, not want to ask anything. 'I know I'm going to die, but my way of coping is to put it at the back of my mind and not to think about it.'

It is easy to fall into the trap of thinking of communication as though it were one way, from adults to children, with factual content only. In fact it is always two way, for even if an adult gives some information to a child there will be some feedback from the child's response.

What is more there is a need for everyone to communicate feelings as well as facts. At one level feelings can best be got across by non-verbal means, the hug that means so much. Feelings can sometimes be expressed only in words: 'I'm not worried about myself when I die, it's my mum and dad I worry about, who's going to look after them?'

Communication systems within the family

Just as one must acknowledge the child's developmental level, so we should respect the existing communication system within the family.

Working with a family where communication is open seems simple: if there is an expectation that people are candid in what they say, whatever the topic, then those matters concerning illness and death will form part of the same pattern. While this is so, even the most open of all families will require an awareness on the part of adults to pick up all the cues that children may give. Christopher's parents held nothing back and their verbal and non-verbal communication with their 6 year old son was a model of how to do it. But towards the end he turned to drawings as a means of communicating, producing pictures with the theme of a small object being guarded and protected by larger ones. Through a careful observation of his drawings and the stories he told to accompany them his parents tuned in to his fears.

Not all families are like this, many deliberately set out to hide facts and feelings from children. The notion of mutual pretence has been discussed by Bluebond-Langner (1978): parents pretend they are not concerned because they do not want to worry their children and children pretend they are not worried because they do not want to upset their parents. As one 10 year old put it, 'I've got to be strong because my mum's had one nervous breakdown and if she thinks I'm cracking she'll have another.'

There are two ways of tackling the problem presented by such a system. One is to go for it headlong: if one confronts the parents openly with the suggestion that they may be using this approach they will often agree that they are. It is then possible, with parental permission, to take this up with the child and thus to allow parents and child to communicate with an adult while retaining the mutual pretence between each other. To accusations of collusion one can respond that this compromise frees both parents and children to communicate in ways that may be, for them, the best possible.

The second approach is to offer opportunities to children to communicate obliquely. Teachers and play specialists have a particular role to play here for the form of communication is often through play or via a school lesson. Robert was a bright 10 year old with leukaemia; he had known several children on his ward die but he had been told by his parents that his illness was not serious. He asked the ward teacher if he could do a project, she replied that she would help in any way she could. The project he chose was blood, a topic allowing him ample opportunity to ask all the questions he needed to.

The families whose system is total avoidance present the hardest problems of all for they will not acknowledge even the notion of mutual pretence. For them the least said, by anyone, the better. While it is not difficult to understand and appreciate at times the value of defence mechanisms, it can be infuriating for professionals who can see the unmet needs on both sides. The oblique opportunities mentioned above may be a solution but even they can be blocked by some parents. A direct confrontation may help but it is more likely than not to lead to further barriers being erected. One approach to effect change is to encourage such parents to join a group when it is possible for other parents to put forward views which may be challenging but which will be perceived as more valid because they come from people with experience. An alternative is to use videos of other families talking about the value of open communication, an example being the film *Over the Rainbow* produced by Maureen Hitcham at the Royal Victoria Infirmary, Newcastle upon Tyne (see p. 62).

Children's concepts of death

There is now an extensive literature on the child's concept of death, mostly from within a Judeo-Christian tradition (Schilder and Wechsler 1934; Nagy 1948; Gartley and Bernasconi 1967; Anthony 1971; Koocher 1973; Melear 1973; Blum 1975; Swain 1975; Kane 1979; McWhirter 1980; Wass and Towry 1980; Reilly *et al.* 1983; Lansdown and Benjamin 1985; Orbach *et al.* 1985). Misra (personal communication) working in India found some responses that would be expected from a different belief system, references to reincarnation, for example.

The concept is complex; children do not go to bed one night knowing nothing about death and wake up next morning knowing everything. One reason for the gradual development of understanding is that the concept itself has at least nine, possibly ten components.

Kane (1979) discusses these components, listing them as shown in Table 10.1, with the ages at which they were attained in her sample. It should be noted that these were American, middle-class children questioned in the late 1970s. As is suggested below, the ages given may not be valid for children in other cultures or, indeed, in America today.

A tenth component is that of personification, the idea of a death figure which comes to take one away. Kane (1979) did not find this in her study; others, for example Nagy (1948), have. I have also found it in clinical practice, when children have nightmares about monsters coming to bear them off.

The development of the concept

It is more or less agreed that children go through stages of understanding, from none to partial to complete, from the concrete to the abstract, from the global to ideas of greater complexity. Typically a 2 year old will not be able to grasp the essential components of the concept, while a 4 year old may know that death means separation but may not realize that it is permanent or that a dead person is unable to see, hear, or move.

Table 10.1 Components of the concept of death

1. Realization	All 3 year olds
2. Separation	5 years
3. Immobility	5 years
4. Irrevocability	6 years
5. Causality	6 years
6. Dysfunctionality	6 years
7. Universality	7 years
8. Insensitivity	8 years
9. Appearance	12 years

From Kane (1979).

Four year old George Sand, told one day that his father had been killed, came down to breakfast next morning to ask, 'Is papa still dead today?'

Lawrence was 5 years old. He had been talking about all sorts of things while playing one of those interminable games of cars that 5 year olds like so much. In the middle of his chatter he suddenly said that he had powers like Jesus. His powers, he went on to explain, enabled him to bring people back from the dead. When asked if he could bring his granny back from the dead he paused and replied that he could not do that because she did not know about his powers.

This episode took place just after Easter and it was clear that Lawrence was trying to assimilate the Easter story into his overall concept.

A number of studies other than that by Kane have attempted to establish the age at which some or all of these components emerge. Lansdown and Benjamin (1985) used a story of an old lady who died in order to tap the understanding of British children aged 5–9 years in London and Essex. Having read the story they then asked the children a series of questions (for example, can the lady come back from being dead?) enabling them to assign a death comprehension score to each child. The results of this study are shown in Table 10.2.

Clunies-Ross and Lansdown (1988) replicated the Lansdown and Benjamin (1985) study using children with leukaemia as subjects. Overall the results were similar to those obtained from healthy children, but there were large individual differences reported.

Two of the key components of the concept, from a clinical point of view, are separation and irrevocability. Once children realize that death means separation there is much to work on. Matthew was almost 5 years when he told his mother that he had bad dreams, about dying. He said that they upset him, 'because I shall miss you and daddy'.

The idea of returning from the dead is common in children of this age (it is, of course, not uncommon in adults). Matthew had another

Table 10.2   Children showing complete or almost complete concepts of death by age

Years	5	6	7	8	9
%	59	73	67	100	96

Adapted from Lansdown and Benjamin (1985).

conversation with his mother a few days before he died. He began by saying that he did not want to be an angel. He went on:

Doctors can't make everyone better, can they.

No but they try very hard.

They can't make me better. But Jesus will make me better with love and kisses because Jesus doesn't give pricks. Then he'll send me back to you and daddy.

It is always as well to remind ourselves that it is dangerous to generalize readily from the averages of a research paper to any one child. We can, nevertheless, come to some cautious conclusions. The first is that children often know more than most adults think they do. The second is that one can be reasonably certain that by 8 or 9 years all children of normal intelligence will have a fully developed idea but we should not forget that many have a good understanding much younger than this.

Concepts of heaven

Six year old Christopher said that when you die you go to heaven, 'where there is more life'. The fact that he had this idea was a great comfort to his parents after his death, underlying the need to know what children know.

The concept of heaven or some other belief about an afterlife, is just as important as that of death in day to day work with children, for they may have some belief, even if there has been no teaching of religion at home. An extreme example was that of Georgina, a 6 year old whose parents were firm atheists who had forbidden any religious instruction in school. When told she was likely to die soon she immediately assumed she would go to heaven and complained to her mother that she would be lonely there. 'Will you', she asked, 'be able to visit me in heaven like you visited me in hospital?'

Despite the readiness with which adults invoke heaven when talking to children about the death of a loved one or a pet, there has been little attempt to discover what children think heaven is like, where it is, how one gets there and so on. A number of studies (Koocher 1973; Melear 1973; Blum 1975; Swain 1975; McWhirter 1980) have asked children what they think happens after death but there have been surprisingly few follow-up probes to investigate what children think in detail.

Frangoulis *et al.* (1996) studied 103 children aged 5–8 years in three London schools. There were differences between responses from two schools which were religious foundations and the third, secular school but these did not reach statistical significance. Well over half declared some belief in heaven but some even of the younger ones were adamant in denying the notion.

Some people do believe in heaven ... yes. But I don't believe it and I'm certain it doesn't happen ... what can happen in a dead body, there is nothing special in it (a 6 year old).

Twenty-five per cent of those who talked of heaven spontaneously mentioned hell. In many cases there were links between the two places.

The oldest person in heaven protects the people ... If someone comes up to heaven by mistake and he's supposed to go to hell, well then they've got to be protected (a 7 year old).

Children facing death not infrequently ask how they will get to heaven. The answers to this question were overwhelmingly in the category of flying or floating up to the sky.

God picks you up—you have to wait 12 days for a flight and then the flight takes 8 hours (a 5 year old).

Only two children who believed in an afterlife were uncertain about the characteristics of the place that people go to. Forty-two per cent thought it more or less like earth as we know it.

They just do normal things that humans do. The children go to school, the older people go to work and the retired ones go to the pub (an 8 year old).

The remaining 56 per cent saw it differently: 43 per cent saw it as pleasant and 36 per cent as unpleasant, sometimes rather frightening, with the rest neutral or uncertain. Heaven is not always a place where much happens, either; 46 per cent reported people there as active and 43 per cent as passive.

Everything is brown, different shades of brown ... because all the people arrive in their coffins and their coffins are brown (a 6 year old).

Heaven has no sound, the sound it has is the sound of the wind and the rain and thunder (a 7 year old).

It has a worrying feel because people might lie and have bad dreams (a 7 year old).

Heaven is a fun place for old people (a 7 year old).

Heaven is not a nice place, lots of animals, red like blood 'cos people have died and have blood. Looks like a dungeon. Feels sad (an 8 year old).

A small number were clearly concerned about overcrowding.

Heaven is 1000 metres big ... if it gets full they will have to give them somewhere else. Another Jesus in another country. Jesus takes them to the other heaven by carriage' (a 6 year old).

Some saw heaven as a place to be made better.

... in the sky is God and God makes them better (a 6 year old).

Forty-nine per cent of those who believed in an afterlife said there is no return. Almost 20 per cent said that one can return from heaven or wherever one is, in human form. Fourteen per cent said that one can visit, 6 per cent asserted that the dead return as ghosts, and a handful mentioned reincarnation in some form or other.

One interviewer probed on dreams and their function and found that 32 per cent of her sample who believed in an afterlife also believed that it is possible for the living to communicate with the dead via their dreams.

Klink (1972) concluded her book on children and religion by hoping that it would be a challenge to psychologists and educationalists to address themselves to the theme of 'the child and faith'. The most striking conclusions from the data presented here are that this topic remains a challenge.

The clinical implications for people working with bereaved children or those who are themselves facing death, their siblings and their parents are evident: we should not assume that 'Gone to heaven' is an answer in itself; it may raise many problems which could need some time to unravel.

Children's concept of the stages of their illness

Along with the acknowledgement that children vary in their understanding of death and the afterlife, so we should try to come to terms with their understanding of their illness. Here the differences are not so much between a full and a partial understanding, rather there are stages of understanding which follow the chronology of the illness.

Ideas fall into five stages.

1. I am ill. For some children, those with cancer, for example, there is a more or less clear-cut beginning to the illness although there may be a grey period before the diagnosis. For others, with a progres-

sive disease, for example, the realization is likely to be more gradual but it is eventually reached.

2. I have an illness that can kill people. Some children reach this stage simply because they hear a word like leukaemia and know perhaps rather vaguely that it is associated with death. Others are told by their parents, if for no other reason than to help explain why the treatment given is so awful. 'If you don't have this you'll die.'

   But it is possible that some children do not believe what they are told. After all, mum said last week that if I didn't tidy my bedroom she'd kill me but she didn't really mean it. It is only when stage 3 is reached that the full realization sinks in.

3. I have an illness that can kill children. When there are three boys with cystic fibrosis in a school one summer term and only two in the autumn, the remaining two have had the clearest possible lesson. We should always be on guard for the ripples that come to a ward or class when a death occurs.

4. I am never going to get better. This may follow on quite quickly after stage 3 and it may take some time. It is almost always associated with depression, a resignation to the continuance of the present state, whatever that may be. It does not, however, imply that children know that their death is imminent. That comes with stage 5.

5. I am going to die. Some authors, for example Bluebond-Langner (1978), argue that all children from approximately 3 years upwards reach this stage. In fact, the hypothesis is untestable and one cannot make this generalization. One must, however, always be on guard for even young children have a full understanding not only of death but of their death.

These five stages give some guidelines about the content of the communication that can be expected to occur.

The key to it all is honesty. In stages 1 and 2, facts are critical.

Felicity was 12 years when a life-threatening illness was diagnosed. She was living with her parents abroad. Her father gave up his job, sold their house, and the whole family moved to London so that she could have medical care. Her parents insisted that she be told nothing more than that she had bad influenza. Felicity herself communicated her needs by screaming after a couple of days, 'You're lying ... you must tell me the truth, you must.'

Learning about the severity of the illness will depend very largely on the nature of the condition. Once children have reached stage 3 and know that their illness can kill children, the focus should be more on what the child communicates to us, rather than vice versa.

Christopher, who has already been quoted, was asked about dying when he was 5 years. He had a form of cancer which meant that the chances of survival were slim and his parents wanted to know what he knew and what he believed so that they could communicate with him as well as possible. In answer to the question, he replied that he was going to be an air force pilot when he grew up and that he would die when his plane was shot down. The message we took away from that conversation was that this was not the right time to open up the topic of his death, rather we were still at the stage of brisk optimism.

At this time and during stages 4 and 5 comes the question of whether or not to tell children that they will die. This is dealt with in more detail below, for the moment the overall rule is that if death is not imminent then it is generally better to act as if a cure is expected or, in cases where the children know there is no cure, as if death is far, far in the future. To tell a child that he or she may die within the next few years is to raise anxiety rather than to allay it.

When death approaches

A question that can cause immense difficulty is whether and when to tell a child that death is near. As mentioned already, some authorities argue that children even as young as 3 years know anyway, while on the other hand many parents are aghast at the idea of telling children because it will worry them. Five points should be kept in mind.

The first is that if children have been given full information about their treatment and the nature of their illness then suddenly to stop telling the truth is likely to arouse considerable anxiety. What, the children may wonder, is happening to me? Why won't anyone explain why dad keeps taking photos of me? Why is aunty Mary here, she had a row with my mum 5 years ago and they never speak to each other? Am I going to have my leg cut off, like the girl in the next bed? Am I going to have my head cut off?

The long term effects *on parents* of not telling the truth can also be considerable.

Max deteriorated suddenly at home and was rushed to hospital. As he was carried into the ambulance he asked his father if he was dying.

His father had not before talked about the possibility of death and, thrown by the question, answered that he would not. Max died in the ambulance and many months afterwards his father castigated himself because, in his words, 'My last words to my son were a lie.'

The third point to bear in mind is that children often indicate by a change in mood that they are preoccupied with an anxiety about something. This change is usually in the direction of becoming withdrawn, in extreme cases stopping talking, eating, and playing. At times like this children are giving a clear message that something is worrying them; they need an opportunity to open up their worries further.

The fourth point is that both what is said and the all important follow-up will depend on the age, understanding, and beliefs of the child. Three year olds often benefit not from talk of death but from reassurance that there will always be someone to look after them. Slightly older children usually take the imminent possibility of death relatively calmly (one 7 year old said 'I'd rather not' as though talking about playing football). My explanation for this is that they see death as a journey, rather just as they have gone from home to school, from one school to another, so they see themselves going on somewhere else.

This makes the assumption that young children facing death all believe in an afterlife and that has, indeed, been my experience. The research quoted above does not bear this out, but that study was carried out on healthy children.

But no matter how calm children may appear to be, there may be anxieties underneath; they may need the opportunity to talk through the implications of what is to happen to them.

As children near their teens so there may be more fear and more anger. This does not mean that death should be denied, only that the same care be taken in offering further chances to talk.

The fifth point is that children should be given the opportunity to talk once they know about their death but they should not be forced to. They should be given a door which they can open or close.

Finally, it is advocated that children be told not that they are going to die, rather that they may die soon. The reason for this is simply that we do not always know that a child will die; even the most expert medical prediction can turn out to be wrong. 'There, I cheated you, didn't I?', said a 14 year old, 'I didn't die after all.'

See also Chapter 5 on communication, Chapter 14 on counselling, and Chapter 19 on staff stress.

References

Anthony, S. (1971). *The discovery of death in childhood and after*. Allen Lane, The Penguin Press, London.

Bluebond-Langner, M. (1978). *The private worlds of dying children*. Princeton University Press, Princeton, NJ.

Blum, A.H. (1975). Children's conceptions of death and an afterlife. *Dissertation Abstracts International*, 36 (10-B), 5248.

Clunies-Ross, C. and Lansdown, R. (1988). The concept of death in children with leukaemia. *Child: Care, Health and Development*, 14, 373–86.

Frangoulis, S., Jordan, N., and Lansdown, R. (1996). Children's concepts of heaven. *British Journal of Religious Education*. (In press.)

Gartley, W. and Bernasconi, M. (1967). The concept of death in children. *Journal of Genetic Psychology*, 110, 71–85.

Kane, B. (1979). Children's concepts of death. *Journal of Genetic Psychology*, 134, 141–53.

Klink, J. (1972). *Your child and religion*. SCM Press, London.

Koocher, G. (1973). Childhood, death and cognitive development. *Developmental Psychology*, 9, 369–75.

Lansdown, R. and Benjamin, G. (1985). The development of the concept of death in children aged 5–9 years. *Child: Care, Health and Development*, 11, 13–20.

McWhirter, L. (1980). *Awareness of death in Belfast children*. Paper presented at the Annual Conference of the British Psychological Society, University of Aberdeen.

Melear, J.D. (1973). Children's conceptions of death. *Journal of Genetic Psychology*, 123, 359–60.

Mullholland, C. (1973). *I'll dance with the rainbows*. Partick Press, Glasgow.

Nagy, N.H. (1948). The child's theories concerning death. *Journal of Genetic Psychology*, 72, 3–27.

Orbach, I., Gross, Y., Glaubman, H., and Berman, D. (1985). Children's perception of death in humans and animals as a function of age, anxiety and cognitive ability. *Journal of Child Psychology and Psychiatry*, 26, 453–63.

Reilly, T.P., Hasazi, J.E., and Bond, L.E. (1983). Children's conceptions of death and personal mortality. *Journal of Pediatric Psychology*, 8, 21–31.

Schilder, P. and Wechsler, D. (1934). The attitudes of children towards death. *Journal of Genetic Psychology*, 45, 406–51.

Swain, H.L. (1975). The concept of death in children. *Dissertation Abstracts International*, 37 (2-A), 898–9.

Wass, H. and Towry, B. (1980). Children's death concepts and ethnicity. *Death Education*, 4, 83–7.

Further reading

Goldman, A. (ed.) (1994). *Care of the dying child.* Oxford University Press, Oxford.

Lansdown, R. and Goldman, A. (1988). The psychological care of children with malignant disease. *Journal of Child Psychology and Psychiatry,* **29,** 555–7.

Pettle Michael, S. and Lansdown, R. (1986). Adjustment to the death of a sibling. *Archives of Disease in Childhood,* **61,** 278–83.

Spinetta, J.J. and Deasy-Spinetta, P. (ed.) (1981). *Living with childhood cancer.* C.V.Mosby, St Louis.

Wass, H. and Corr, C.A. (ed.) (1984). *Childhood death.* Hemisphere Publishing Corporation, Washington.

Wells, R. (1988). *Helping children cope with grief.* Sheldon Press, London.

11

Body and mind

This is the great error of our day, that physicians separate the mind from the body (Plato).

Despite Plato, entrenched positions on the nature of the mind–body relationship are still not uncommon. On the one hand, we have the extreme, reductionist, so-called medical model which looks only to signs of disease and only to organically based cures. To someone following this line it makes no difference who or what the patient is, thinks, or hopes. At the other extreme is the person who looks to the mind not only as a causal factor in all illness but also as something which can, if harnessed properly, cure practically everything.

A more balanced view is that we have to look to both mind and body if we are to understand fully any illness, on the understanding that at times one influence will be more powerful than the other.

Some definitions

'Psychosomatic', was coined in 1818 by the German psychiatrist Heinioth when describing insomnia (Margetts 1950). It refers to the inseparability and interdependence of psychosocial and biological aspects of humankind and was originally used to mean just that, that is to cut across the dichotomy between diagnoses as either physical (somatic) or psychological. When the *Journal of Psychosomatic Medicine* was founded in 1939 its stated aim was to study in their interrelation the psychological and physical aspects of all normal and abnormal bodily functions.

Diseases can be designated as psychosomatic if two conditions are fulfilled.

1. There are demonstrable physiological disturbances of function.

2. The illness as a whole can be interpreted as a manifestation or function of the patient's personality, conflicts, or life style (Rycroft 1987).

From this one could say that the proper focus of study is the person, not the disease. Unfortunately, some diseases have, nevertheless, gained a label of 'psychosomatic', which means in practice that conditions like atopic dermatitis, bronchial asthma, and gastric ulcers came to be seen as 'all in the mind'. Perhaps because it has been misunderstood, perhaps because no distinctive psychosomatic process has been identified, it is now falling out of fashion: two recently published books on child psychiatry (Graham 1991; Black and Cottrell 1993) do not include the word in their indexes.

'Psychogenic' means having a psychological origin, it is usually used for factors related to a condition.

'Psychosocial' refers to interdependent psychological and social factors.

'Somatoform disorders' are those conditions in which there is a tendency to experience psychological states as bodily sensations, functional changes, or somatic metaphors (Lipowski 1967). They come in two main types: in the first patients perceive a physical disorder to be present despite the absence of any evidence for an illness and, in the second, sometimes known as conversion disorders, physical symptoms, such as paralysis, exist without any evidence of an underlying disease.

Stress as a causal factor in illness

Tohru Ishigami, of Osaka, Japan, wrote in the *American Review of Tuberculosis* that the key to the understanding of that illness lies in the emotional life of the patient. The article was published in 1919 but it is only in the last decade or so that there has come an influential and increasing interest in the role of stress and emotions in the cause and maintenance of illness. As one author has put it, 'When stocks go down in New York, diabetes goes up' (DRD 1987).

The immune system, hitherto thought to be closed, is now commonly linked with the nervous system, each exercising some control over the other. A popular account of the discoveries related to this new discipline of studying the mind, the nervous system, and the immune system, a discipline known as psychoneuroimmunology, is given by Locke and Colligan (1986). To take just three examples they quote:

1. The immune systems of depressed people are less responsive than those of normal controls or others suffering from different mental illnesses.

2. University students who failed to cope with the stress of examinations had depressed immunological responses when compared with those who coped well.

3. Cancer cells injected into rats produced tumours twice as often in animals that had been stressed by electric shocks into a state of helplessness than others. The standard academic text is that of Ader *et al.* (1991).

Biological vulnerability

Animal work on the effects of stress tends to produce a pattern in which the type of stress is related to the physical outcome; in humans the picture is more complex and seems to indicate that there is a more or less fixed pattern to each patient. In other words, there is a predisposition to a disease, whatever the psychological factors (Gregg 1983). Evidence from children suggests that the pattern of organ vulnerability is laid down by the age of 6 years (DRD 1987).

Personality characteristics

There has been some attempt to link the inability to express emotions in words with the tendency towards somatization but it could be argued that this is a function of culture and/or family patterns rather than personality as such. There is no evidence for an association between personality types being associated with particular conditions. The idea of the asthmatic personality, for example, is not tenable.

Perpetuating factors

A condition may have cause A but be maintained by factor B. An example often cited in this context is the post-viral fatigue syndrome or myalgic encephalopathy (ME). People seem to have had a viral illness but then some of them take months or even years to recover their former vigour. Graham, quoted in Lask and Fosson (1989) refers to another type of ME to explain at least some of these cases: manipulative emotionality. He sees such children as having a degree of control over their behaviour for they are often very much better when adults are not present. Detailed questioning usually reveals school or family difficulties.

Another, similar phenomenon is that referred to as the high achieving syndrome. Similar in presentation to ME, this involves children who have been well behaved, high achievers at school, popular with peers, from happy and well functioning families. One explanation is that the fatigue gives a good reason for retreating from an over-demanding world, the children concerned seeming to be those who cannot bear to fail and who could never express negative feelings towards their parents.

Children

A high proportion of the relatively few studies that have been carried out with children have focused on diabetes. Johnson (1988) reviewed the literature and pointed out that in the seventeenth century the disease was seen as the result of 'prolonged sorrow'. She went on to examine the interaction between the disease, the patient, and the environmental context within which the child lives, concluding that while one can say that there are effects of one on the others it is very difficult to specify the exact linkages involved. Some disorders in which there is often evidence of mind and body implications are discussed below.

Conversion disorders

Hypochondriasis and other forms of disturbed self-perception of illness are rare in childhood and more common in adolescence, but conversion disorders, which used to be called hysterical disorders, are more frequent in childhood. Conversion is said to occur when an emotional conflict is transformed into a physical disability. It may be no more than a way of avoiding an unwanted experience, when there is some secondary gain, or it may have symbolic significance, like a weakness in one's hand associated with emotions related to aggression. Children can then be seen to enjoy the benefits of taking on the sick role, within the framework of illness behaviour.

Abdominal pain

Between 10 and 20 per cent of schoolchildren experience recurrent abdominal pain but only 1 in 20 have a known organic cause (Apley *et al.* 1978). Pain may occur daily for hours at a time or much less regularly. It is rarely reported at night; if it does a primary organic cause is most likely.

Many other terms, seen by Lask and Fosson (1989) as euphemisms, have been used to describe this condition, including irritable bowel syndrome, abdominal migraine, spastic colon, periodic syndrome, and cyclical vomiting. In fact, periodic syndrome should be kept for those children who have recurrent episodes of abdominal pain, headache, and vomiting, while cyclical vomiting should be reserved for those who have recurrent episodes of dramatic vomiting often leading to dehydration.

Other pain syndromes

These can include pains in the head, chest, limbs, and joints and are generally similar to abdominal pain in nature. Limb pains affect one in five children, rarely with an established organic cause (Apley *et al.* 1978) and one in seven have headaches, of whom two-thirds may have no detected physical abnormalities (Jerrett 1979). There is no support for the notion that growing pains have much to do with physical growth (Naish and Apley 1951).

Asthma

Asthma, the commonest chronic physical disorder in childhood, seems to be increasing in frequency. There is commonly a family history of allergic disorder and children suffering from the illness have often had an episode of infantile eczema.

Psychological factors may be of great importance in bringing about attacks and in maintaining them but the earlier-held view that this is an illness primarily of a psychological nature is now no longer held. There is no clearly defined 'asthmatic personality' and no evidence that environmental events play a part in the aetiology of the condition.

Some children, however, learn how to bring on attacks, perhaps to avoid unwanted activity or to draw attention to themselves and/or away from others. Approximately, 10 per cent of asthmatic children show significant emotional and behavioural problems and have a higher rate of disturbance than healthy controls (Mrazek *et al.* 1987). In this they are, of course, no different from other children with chronic conditions, a point discussed above.

Bladder and bowel disorders

It is well-known fact that children not infrequently wet the bed when they first come into hospital, an indication of stress. Daytime wetting is usually a sign of more serious disturbance.

Constipation may be related to a clear organic condition, Hirsch-sprung's disease, for example, or epidermolysis bullosa, and there must always be a very careful physical examination before treatment begins.

Encopresis, sometimes defined as the depositing of formed faeces in inappropriate places, sometimes used more generally to refer to any soiling, is a different matter for while there are possible physical causes involved there is a higher chance that psychosocial factors will be relevant. Confusion can be caused with constipation since the latter can cause soiling by overflow.

Anorexia nervosa

This involves a determined food avoidance, usually but not always in girls, frequently observed at the time of the expected growth spurt. The clinical picture can be confused with depression, cyclical vomiting, or school phobia. Whatever the cause(s) in individual cases, there is no doubt that a multidisciplinary approach, bringing in physicians and a psychosocial team, is essential for treatment.

Obesity and overeating

Of all the conditions mentioned in this chapter obesity is one of the hardest to combat. Approximately 10 per cent of children may be affected, from all social classes. There is commonly a family pattern of overeating with habits being instilled early in life. One approach is to perceive overeating as an addiction: despite the frequent claims by parents and others that 'it's all glandular', there is rarely any evidence to support an underlying, simple biological explanation.

Tics and Tourette's syndrome

Tics are sudden, involuntary, and purposeless muscle movements. Most often affected are the face, head, and neck. Tourette's syndrome is rare (fewer than 1 in a 1000) and involves complex tics, vocalizations, and, even more embarrassingly, swearing.

More boys than girls are affected by tics. It is thought that there is probably a combination of factors leading to tics, including genetic influences, neurological abnormalities, and undue stress. One of the first tasks in treatment is to assess possible causes of anxiety.

Psychogenic coughs can be treated in the same way as tics.

Migraine

In childhood, migraine is rarely diagnosed before the age of 9 or 10 years. It typifies the futility of the either–or approach, as factors that may need to be taken into account include diet, exercise, and stress. Treatment can involve both medication and relaxation techniques.

Management

Although each set of symptoms requires a particular approach, there are some common threads to management. Taking a very careful history can often reveal some of the factors leading to the problems and observation of the child with and without significant adults can be illuminating in seeing how behaviour varies according to whoever is around reinforcing certain patterns. Even examining doctors can find themselves unwittingly rewarding children for illness behaviour by showing such an interest in their condition. Next comes the need to try to see the picture from the point of view of the family. Challenging them with 'It's all in her mind' or even worse, that 'It's all the parents' fault' is apt to be counter-productive. Better to share with the family that while no causes for the symptoms have been found there is no suggestion that the child is putting it on; rather there has to be a partnership in which the professionals and the parents start from a position of being mystified about the physical cause. The next step is to suggest strongly that recovery will occur within a short period, a few weeks perhaps, and the child should be told to expect increasing improvement and control. It may help to give children a chance to recover with honour; using physiotherapy or hypnosis are two ways of helping recovery to occur without a loss of face.

A major hazard

A particular hazard is that some people see stress at the root of all ill-nesses and then look to stress-reducing activities as a cure for even the most serious condition. This approach, which has occasionally been used for children, can be harmful. A boy of 12 years, with cancer, was upset when he relapsed not only because this meant more treatment but because he imagined that his attempts at relaxation had not been good enough.

Conclusion

As Lask and Fosson (1989) have stated, in practice virtually all disorders have multifactorial causation. The factors include developmental, biological, social, and psychological. Totman (1989) concluded that recent research has made it clear that the risk of becoming seriously ill is affected more profoundly by social factors than by physical wear and tear. Even the most conservative would, today, probably allow that psychosocial factors are involved in a vast majority of illnesses.

Lask and Fosson (1989) make much of an anonymous author who wrote of the psychosomatic approach being a matter of listening to children talking with their bodies. It is a fine way of summarizing the two major strands of mind and body that are so often so difficult to disentangle.

References

Ader, R., Felton, D.L., and Cohen, N. (1991). *Psychoneuroimmunology*, (2nd edn). Academic Press, San Diego.

Apley, J., MacKeith, R., and Meadow, R. (1978). *The child and his symptoms: a comprehensive approach*. Blackwell, Oxford.

Black, D. and Cottrell, D. (ed.) (1993). *Seminars in child and adolescent psychiatry*. Gaskell, London.

DRD (1987). Psychosomatic disease: a medical view. In *The Oxford companion to the mind*, (ed. R.L. Gregory). Oxford University Press, Oxford.

Graham, P. (1991). *Child psychiatry: a developmental approach*, (2nd edn). Oxford University Press, Oxford.

Gregg, I. (1983). Epidemiological aspects. In *Asthma* (2nd edn) (ed. T.J.H. Clark and S. Godfrey). Chapman & Hall, London.

Jerrett, W. (1979). Headaches in general practice. *Practitioner*, 222, 549–55.

Johnson, S.B. (1988). Diabetes mellitus in childhood. In *Handbook of pediatric psychology*, (ed. D.K. Routh). The Guilford Press, New York.

Lask, B. and Fosson, A. (1989). *Childhood illness: the psychosomatic approach*. John Wiley, Chichester.

Lipowski, Z. (1967). Review of consultation psychiatry and psychosomatic medicine: II. Clinical aspects. *Psychosomatic Medicine*, **29**, 201–24.

Locke, S. and Colligan, D. (1986). *The healer within*. Mentor Books, New York.

Margetts, E.L. (1950). The early history of the word 'psychosomatic'. *Canadian Medical Association Journal*, **63**, 402–5.

Mrazek, D.A., Casey, B., and Anderson, I. (1987). Insecure attachment in severely asthmatic preschool children: is it a risk factor? *Journal of the American Academy of Child and Adolescent Psychiatry*, **26**, 516–20.

Naish, J. and Apley, J. (1951). Growing pains: a clinical study of non-arthritic limb pains in children. *Archives of Disease in Childhood*, **26**, 134–40.

Rycroft, C. (1987). Psychosomatic disease: philosophical and psychological aspects. In *The Oxford companion to the mind*, (ed. R.L. Gregory). Oxford University Press, Oxford.

Totman, P. (1989). *Social causes of illness*. Souvenir Press, London.

12

Munchausen syndrome by proxy

One of the more curious phenomena, one of those findings reported in textbooks that many people find impossible to believe—until they experience it first hand—is a syndrome known as Munchausen syndrome by proxy (MSBP).

The term Munchausen syndrome was first coined in 1951 by Richard Asher when he described a psychiatric disorder in which people fabricate medical histories and conditions in order to gain medical attention. They go from doctor to doctor, from hospital to hospital, often undergoing treatment which is medically quite unwarranted. The syndrome was named after the eighteenth century Baron Karl Fredereick von Munchausen, famous for his grossly exaggerated tales of adventures.

The idea that people might seek medical attention for social reasons was, however, known well before 1951. The *London Daily News* of 18 May 1870 carried a report on the new hospital in Shoreditch, later to become Queen Elizabeth Hospital, Hackney. It was noted that there was a charge (of two pence) because

At great free hospitals it is known that a large number of the cases presenting from treatment are absolutely free from ailments. A gossip with the patients waiting, the factitious importance of being examined and questioned by the doctor, a morbid pleasure in attending at the hospital and in showing a large bottle of medicine to the admiring neighbours up the narrow court—these are the inducements which convert many a poor ignorant woman into a malade imaginaire.

The 'proxy' was added by Roy Meadow in 1977 to apply by extension to the parent or caretaker who needs to have a sick child. Such parents, more usually mothers than fathers, often have some medical knowledge and know how to produce the results. In extreme cases they will administer noxious substances to their children to make them ill; in very extreme cases the children die (Rosenberg 1987; Meadow 1989).

The number of reported cases has increased dramatically in Britain in the last decade (Bools *et al.* 1992) and as the numbers have risen so has the sophistication of the description of the syndrome. It is not 'a specific entity with a specific cause requiring a specific line of management' (Meadow 1984) rather it is 'a complicated phenomenon whereby a threefold relationship between perpetrator, victim and medical staff develops' (Sigal *et al.* 1989). It can also be seen as an unusual form of child abuse.

Warning signals

There is a strong possibility of Munchausen syndrome by proxy and the hospital's social services department should be alerted immediately in the case of the following.

1. If a child presents with illnesses for which a cause cannot readily be found.

2. If the illness is persistent over time and results in social and/or physical disability.

3. If there are inconsistencies in test results.

4. If the parent is markedly attentive to the child's needs, reluctant to be parted from the child, insisting that she is the only one from whom the child will accept food or medication.

5. If the parent is highly involved in the medical care of the other children on the ward.

6. If the father is not involved in medical decisions, even if they be of importance.

7. If the parent welcomes more and more tests.

8. If the child's symptoms reduce when apart from the parent.

Reported cases

Reports on MSBP cover an age range from infancy to adolescence with the duration lasting up to 4 years. Children have been poisoned, most commonly with domestic salt, and drugs have been administered orally, rectally, and even via naso-gastric or intravenous tubes. Charts can be tampered with, specimens can be doctored, and very young children may even be suffocated (Samuels *et al.* 1992). Other symptoms have included rashes produced by scratches and failure to thrive caused by the withholding of food or induced vomiting.

One of the commonest forms of MSBP is fictitious epilepsy (Meadow 1991), the symptoms of which can be taught by a parent and were, in one case, to a child as young as 4 years.

Older children may join with the perpetrating adult in producing and maintaining symptoms, even in one extreme case, a child with normal limbs, who was confined to a wheelchair with imagined spina bifida (Meadow 1985).

Children suffering from what is sometimes called MUPS (medically undiagnosed physical symptoms) are often given the diagnosis of hysteria, the criteria for which are some model for sickness, real or contrived, an ally (usually a parent or parents), and the necessary social skill to present the symptoms (Taylor 1986).

The line between hysteria and MSBP is fine and the two diagnoses may not be mutually exclusive.

Characteristics of the parent

In reported cases it has almost always been the mother who has been implicated. There has been a wide age range, and a similar wide range in educational levels. The frequency with which mothers have or claim to have some medical or paramedical association is striking, thus explaining the skill with which fabrication can be conducted.

It is enormously difficult to understand the motives of mothers. They may give a highly unreliable history, financial gain is not usually enough to explain their actions, and while no one would argue that they are behaving normally, there is often insufficient evidence otherwise to lead to a diagnosis of psychiatric disorder.

Some mothers have themselves had a history of multiple unexplained illness when younger. It can be postulated that they see their child as needing the same attention that they received at the same age. Others may be escaping from an unhappy marriage or some other daily stress. One interpretation of poisoning was that the mother could not differentiate emotionally between herself and the child and so her own suicidal tendency was expressed.

At least 25 per cent of one series of mothers of suffocated children had themselves been abused when young and 60 per cent of another series had a history of psychiatric disorder in childhood or adolescence.

There is little information on fathers other than the generalization that they apparently spend little time with their families, even when their children are in hospital. If MSBP is found or suspected it is worth considering the status of siblings for there is a high incidence of unexplained infant death or unexplained illness in them (Meadow 1984*a,b*; Bools *et al.* 1992).

Management

Once staff have been alerted to the possibility of MSBP it is vital to try to take a careful history of the parents' illnesses and of the siblings if this has not already been done.

Attention to medical management will depend on the presenting symptoms. It may be necessary to send samples of blood, urine, vomitus, or gastric aspirate for toxicological analysis to see if there is poisoning from drugs available from other members of the family. It may even be necessary to test maternal blood to check that this has not been introduced into a child's sample.

Ultimately it is often essential to separate the mother from the child to observe the subsequent course of the illness. Here it is best to come as close as possible to the truth in explaining the reasons for separation: the mother's presence may in some way be interacting with the child through allergic or emotional factors or as a result of something that they are doing to each other.

A rarely undertaken technique is to video the child and mother without either knowing. The ethics of this approach have been questioned and it must be followed only after discussions with social services and the hospital's ethical committee.

Once there is evidence for MSBP a child protection meeting should be convened by social services, followed by a meeting with the assumed perpetrator to explain the current thinking.

This confrontation is not, of course, to be taken lightly. The most common response from mothers, even after video evidence has been produced, is to deny intent to harm. Suicide threats or attempts are not unknown but while relatively few parents accept the need for psychiatric help, it is essential to involve a member of the psychiatric team in the case from the earliest possible time. Even if the mother refuses therapy the child is likely to need some support once separation has been achieved. This support may involve helping the child to understand, as best anyone can, what has been happening and it may involve enabling the child to switch from the sick role that has been fostered for so long.

Following that meeting the child will need to be in a safe environment and will also need medical care appropriate for what is now seen as the true illness.

The safety of the child having been ensured, there remains the need to decide whether the family can continue to care for that child or any other children. Characteristics thought to be unfavourable for a return of the child to a mother include harm inflicted on a younger child, denial of behaviour, a history of Munchausen syndrome, any history of unexplained death or illness in the family, and significant adverse social settings, for example where there is evidence of serious drug or alcohol abuse.

References

Asher, R. (1951). Munchausen's syndrome. *Lancet*, 339–41.

Bools, C.N., Neale, B.A., and Meadow, R. (1992). Co-morbidity associated with fabricated illness (Munchausen syndrome by proxy). *Archives of Disease in Childhood*, **67**, 77–9.

Meadow, R. (1982). Munchausen syndrome by proxy. *Archives of Disease in Childhood*, **57**, 92–8.

Meadow, R. (1984a). Factitious illness: the hinterland of child abuse. *Recent Advances in Paediatrics*, **7**, 217–32.

Meadow, R. (1984b). Fictitious epilepsy. *Lancet*, **2**, 25–8.

Meadow, R. (1985). Management of Munchausen syndrome by proxy. *Archives of Diseases in Childhood*, **60**, 385–93.

Meadow, R. (1989). Munchausen syndrome by proxy. *British Medical Journal*, **299**, 248–50.

Meadow, R. (1990). Suffocation, recurrent apnea and sudden infant death. *Journal of Paediatrics*, **117**, 351–7.

Meadow, R. (1991). Neurological and developmental variants of Munchausen syndrome by proxy. *Developmental Medicine and Child Neurology*, **33**, 270–2.

Rosenberg, D.A. (1987). Web of deceit: a literature review of Munchausen syndrome by proxy. *Journal of Child Abuse*, **11**, 547–63.

Samuels, M.P., McLaughlin, W., Jacobson, R.R., Poets, C.F., and Southall, D. (1992). Fourteen cases of imposed upper airway obstruction. *Archives of Disease in Childhood*, **67**, 162–70.

Sigal, M., Selkopf, M., and Meadow, R. (1989). Munchausen by proxy syndrome. The triad of abuse, self abuse and deception. *Comprehensive Psychiatry*, **30**, 527–33.

Taylor, D.C. (1986). Hysteria, playacting and courage. *British Journal of Psychiatry*, **149**, 37–41.

13

Cooperation with treatment

A powerful description of what it feels like in a non-compliant phase of diabetes was given in the December 1993 issue of the British Diabetic Association magazine *Balance*:

I felt unable to accept my diabetes. Sometimes it felt like a punishment I deserved and that I must therefore be an awful person but at other times it seemed like a punishment for nothing—an unjust punishment. My reactions to these feelings had been to ignore the fact that I am diabetic and pretend, as much as possible, that I didn't have it. Naturally this resulted in poor control and a refusal to 'behave' in any way which could accommodate diabetes into my life.

More has been written about the psychological aspects of diabetes than almost any other chronic condition, possibly more than any other. The reasons are not difficult to see, since this is one disease whose treatment is so dependent on the compliance of the child and, hence, on the child's frame of mind. Just as there has to be a balance between food and insulin, so there has to be a recognition of the pressures from peers to be ordinary, like everyone else, and from parents and medical staff to pay attention to one's physical state. Diabetes is, however, far from being the only condition touched by the problem.

The extent and nature of the problem

The failure to comply with medical treatment has been described in an American publication as 'A problem of enormous dimension for all health-care providers ... underestimated by physicians and grossly understated by patients.' It carries 'a multibillion dollar price tag and a heavy toll of human suffering' (Rissman and Rissman 1987).

This was written in the context of adult patients but there is evidence enough that the problem exists in children, in adolescents, and in families. La Greca (1988) mentions 15 studies coming to this conclusion, one of which estimated the overall compliance rate to be approximately 50 per cent of the paediatric populations, largely American, reported on.

Definitions

Compliance is usually defined as the extent to which a person's behaviour—in terms of keeping appointments, taking medications, and executing life style changes—coincides with medical advice (Haynes *et al.* 1979). As a term it has been criticized as being authoritarian, implying a one-way relationship between doctor and patient, with adherence or cooperation being preferred, hence the title of this chapter.

Measuring cooperation

There is no evidence that doctors are very good at judging whether a patient has been compliant. Haynes *et al.* (1979) suggest that predictability based on tossing a coin is as good as a physician's opinion.

There are, however, a number of ways of measuring cooperation, reflecting the components in the definition given above. Drug assays, examining blood or urine for drug contents, is one, patient or parent reports another. The former are useful for short periods of treatment but patients can cheat by taking the drug just before the time they know there is going to be a test. The latter are subject to bias and tend towards overestimating cooperation. Observations are a third way that can be effective, depending on who is observing.

Factors associated with cooperation

There is no evidence that age, gender, marital status, personality characteristics, education, or socio-economic status are associated with less cooperation, although chronic conditions requiring long-term treatments are linked with lower rates. The severity of symptoms does not appear to increase cooperation (Rissman and Rissman 1987; Madsen 1992). The evidence that does exist suggests that non-compliance is related to those diseases with a complex treatment régime or those where the child's physical appearance is involved (La Greca 1990).

It would seem that increasing parents' and children's knowledge should significantly improve cooperation rates. Mattar *et al.* (1975) found that in one group of parents only 5 per cent were fully compliant but only 4 per cent fully understood the utility and nature of the medication prescribed. When attention was paid to instructing parents more carefully the compliance rate improved to 51 per cent. However, in the adult literature the association between knowledge and compliance is unclear (Becker and Maiman 1980). One way of interpreting the data available is to see information about the condition and its treatment as necessary but not sufficient.

Dunbar and Stunkard (1979) argue that the treatment regimen itself is 'the single most important determinant of patient adherence'. They see decreases in complexity, duration, requirements for changes in life style, inconvenience, and cost as likely to bring about greater cooperation.

Much of the work relevant to paediatrics is based on family systems models, an example being the model of Harkaway and Madsen (1989) which sees the family and the health care providers as two distinct cultures which come together to form a third. Difficulties in the operation of this system are seen to arise in terms of meaning, which subsumes notions of belief and of action. This reinforces the idea that we should be looking at interactions rather than at obedience. The role of belief is particularly relevant to adolescents, for there may be discrepancies between their health belief model and that held by parents or health care staff.

The are four factors involved in this belief model (Becker 1974).

1. Motivation, by which is meant the degree of interest in and concern about health matters in general.

2. Susceptibility: perceptions of vulnerability to the illness.

3. Severity: perceptions concerning the seriousness of the consequences of contracting an illness or of neglecting its treatment.

4. Benefits and costs, seeing the latter as encompassing inconvenience and loss of face as well as financial debits.

Developmental factors

Early childhood

Developmental patterns and treatment intertwine. For the baby and toddler, parents must be in charge of all tests and treatment. The main problem here is the near impossibility of explaining to a young child why all this is being done. This is especially hard in the case of the child who comes into hospital for planned treatment, feeling quite well, and is then subjected to pain and discomfort. The idea that young children may believe that they are in hospital because they have been naughty is discussed in Chapter 4. If this is the case then those children may perceive treatment as a punishment.

As the child approaches the 'terrible twos' stage resulting from a developing sense of self and competence, the parents often face non-compliance with treatment for the first time. Additionally, parents and extended family often feel the temptation to avoid upsetting the child as compensation for the suffering of the illness. Toddlers then learn that they can manipulate their parents' anxiety to get their own way. This often results in the failure of parents to gain positions of authority, draw family boundaries, and set limits on the children's behaviour. The consequences of such management styles are continued non-compliance with a medical regimen and a general insecurity in those children who have never felt a sense of parental control.

School entrance involves exposure to a wider audience for the illness. It requires explanations, understanding, and, in some cases, unsolicited adverse reactions. A frequent cough and different approach to food can make the child feel with cystic fibrosis different when the normal drive is to be like the others. A sense of isolation and loneliness can lower self-esteem. A child can become withdrawn and watchful or, alternatively, boisterous and aggressive as a means of compensation. Helping the child feel positive about cystic fibrosis, having confidence in providing explanations, and aiding the child participate in normal life experiences are essential.

At school age there is the need to explain the problem to teachers and to trust them to be vigilant. There is the need also to help children cope with their difference, something which they may not before have been aware of. The more popular the child, the worse this may be for there will be more parties, with sweet food, to contend with.

Middle childhood

In middle childhood issues tend to concern the children themselves and are similar to those of other diseases. They are able to understand the nature of their illness and a need to incorporate cystic fibrosis, for example, into their personal identity. They need permission to be themselves rather than the illness taking priority. Providing accurate, honest information is essential with this age group. Parents who lie will have great difficulty maintaining trustworthy relationships as the child discovers the truth.

With diabetes, the particular source of conflict in the middle school years is to do with dietary control but it is the transfer of responsibility for insulin injections that causes most anxiety. Children commonly learn to give their own injections by 8 or 9 years and should be capable of independent management, including testing their urine for sugar, by 11 or 12 years.

Particular problems often concern adherence to diet, cooperation with physiotherapy, needle phobia, how to tell school, and dealing with being teased.

The children often face the dilemma of requiring a large calorie intake but having no interest in food. One child described 'never being excited by food like other people'. Each mealtime can be aversive and akin to force feeding; food, rather than a source of pleasure, is seen as part of a medical routine.

Physiotherapy takes time away from other preferable activities and is a reminder of the illness. It also, often, involves parents and so requires timetabling for the family and cooperative relationships.

Adolescence

Issues of compliance loom at this time; non-compliance rates in adolescents are generally considered higher than among other age groups (Eiser 1993). But it is not enough to dismiss all adolescent behaviour as part of the normal 'storm and stress' of this period, mainly because the hard evidence to support the notion that adolescents are, as a breed, hell on wheels, simply is not there (Lansdown and Walker 1991). Indeed, the current view is that the linear relationship between age and compliance is to be called into question (Eiser 1973).

The beginning of secondary education can, indeed, often coincide with a change of personality and a new non-compliance with treatment. At a time of life when most children are expanding their experience, planning their future career, and actively seeking opportunity, children with some illnesses can be contemplating their own mortality.

In some conditions, for example diabetes, the onset of puberty will bring with it physical factors that make the control of an illness more difficult than hitherto. In sick children the psychological (as opposed to the physical) phase of adolescence seems sometimes to begin early. Many parents have talked to me of their ill children having old heads on young shoulders and it appears that the daily management of a chronic and terminal illness can bring a sense of premature self-responsibility and opinions irrespective of intelligence level.

Similar cognitive development to that seen during the toddler stage seems to bring about similar behaviour. A reconsidered sense of self, a capacity for greater competence, and legal self-responsibility can result in splitting from family and rejection of medical opinion.

The strength of peer pressure during this stage of life often introduces potential problems such as teenage pregnancy, smoking, alcohol, and drug abuse. It should also be noted, though, that peers can be very supportive, for example in changing their own eating habits to fit in with those of a diabetic friend.

Family factors

Virtually all families, whatever their cohesiveness, find their routine upset to some extent when a child is in hospital; all children are affected by what is going on in the family. In the context of paediatric care a badly functioning family is of especial importance. Among pre-adolescent children non-cooperation is closely related to family behaviour and even in adolescence this is by no means a minor consideration. In diabetes, for example, there is good evidence that poor relationships, rigidity, and lack of cohesion are associated with poorer metabolic control (Bobrow *et al.* 1985). Unfortunately, the converse is not always true, that is supportive families do not guarantee good control in diabetes, it is more complex than that (Eiser 1993).

It is usually the mother who assumes the major responsibility for ensuring that treatment is carried out when the child is at home but she is only a part of a system. As is discussed below, there is something to be said for approaching a family as such rather than concentrating on a mother–child dyad.

Modifying the system

Ethical issues

It is easy to see why health staff become exasperated with patients who do not take their advice and who do not keep appointments. Yet, while failing an appointment with no warning is ill mannered, there may be support from ethicists for those who feel that people have a right to refuse to follow certain treatment regimes or to have some invasive investigations. Apart from the right to refuse as such, patients may have logic on their side. It may be that the disadvantages in keeping to a strict regime, in terms of cost, inconvenience, and the problems of side-effects, may be seen as marginally greater than what can be gained by adhering fully. After all, following the letter of even the best medical treatment does not always bring full symptom relief. What is more, the doctors may be wrong: today's orthodoxy can be tomorrow's heresy.

To add even more, two recent studies, Close *et al.* (1986) and Fonagy *et al.* (1987), have indicated that there is a price to pay for compliance: children may become depressed in the face of the heavy demands made on them.

Considerations of ethics have led to three pre-conditions for the use of techniques to enhance cooperation.

1. The diagnosis must be correct.

2. The treatment must do more good than harm.

3. The patient (and/or parent) must be an informed, willing partner in the endeavour.

What can be done

The obvious action to take is first of all to ensure that everyone concerned has adequate information and then to harangue parents, children, and grandparents even, so that they get the importance of the treatment into their heads. It is not as easy as that (La Greca 1988); if it were there would be no need to write this chapter.

A second approach is to try to change the health care providers' attitudes and behaviour. Doctors who are brusque, who give little or no feedback to patients, who appear to discount patients' views are seen as central to the problem. In contrast, Francis *et al.* (1969) found that mothers' compliance with a regime prescribed for their children was greater when they felt that the physician was friendly, understood the condition, and was able to explain its cause and treatment. Summarizing the results of studies in this area one can say, not surprisingly, that adherence is greater when patient (or parent) expectations have been fulfilled, when sincere concern is shown, and when the provider and client substantially agree on the specifics of the regime.

One shift in provider behaviour has been shown to improve cooperation: the degree of supervision. Hospitalized patients do better than day patients, who do better than out-patients. Out-patient cooperation can be enhanced with more careful supervision, though: Fink *et al.* (1969) showed a difference of 59 per cent and 18 per cent in compliance in a study of 274 children as a function of the follow-up supervision provided by a nurse.

Behavioural techniques

Self-monitoring, for example, making a note of medicine taken on a calendar, is probably most helpful in cases of acute illness with short-term medication regimes.

Reinforcement procedures involve what psychologists call providing rewards and what parents call bribery. (There is a distinction: a bribe is given for an act which is illegal or immoral.) They too, are likely to be helpful in the case of fairly simple conditions, with short treatment patterns. The more complex the difficulties the less likely it is that behavioural approaches will be effective on their own (La Greca 1986). In conjunction with other techniques they can be of value.

Family therapy and its techniques

Altschuler *et al.* (1991) have described a study of family factors in compliance and treatment and have described in some detail family work with adolescents in end-stage renal failure. Rissman and Rissman (1987) have discussed the use of strategies often employed by family therapists in more general terms, seeing them as valuable in preventing as well as treating non-compliance.

Joining the family system is their starting point. The therapist, in this context the doctor or other health worker, must let the family know that he or she understands them and is working with and for them. Joining is expressing an interest in non-medical aspects of the patient's world and sharing some small element of the doctor's world with the patient.

Avoiding more of the same implies not repeating what has been tried, in vain, already.

Reframing the problem involves altering someone's view of it. A key factor is the need to take into account the views, attitudes, and beliefs of the person. A mother worried that vaccination might harm her baby because something unnatural would be introduced into the body.

She was helped, within the framework of seeing what is natural as good, by an explanation that immunization stimulates the body's own, that is, natural, defences against disease.

Taking a one-down position is recommended when a child or parent has been subjected to a barrage of authoritarian commands. There is nothing like telling some people that they must or must not do something to turn them in the other direction. It may be necessary to tread a fine line here: giving orders from on high does not work but then to appear to abdicate all responsibility and say that all decisions are up to the patient may give the wrong message as well. One of my colleagues gives all sides of the picture and then tells the parents that of course what they choose to do is up to them but that if it were his child he would ...

Predicting partial failure in maintaining a regime is another approach to enable patients to fail with honour. If they are warned that they are being asked to do something difficult and that most people fall down at some time or another, it makes discussing the failures much more comfortable. It helps to explain to parents of a child with diabetes that there is no such thing as a perfectly controlled person any more than there is a perfect parent.

Conclusion

An expert is someone who says, whatever the question, 'It's more complicated than you think.' This is certainly so of the issue discussed in this chapter. There are so many factors involved not only in the nature and cause of the problem but also in the approach to a solution, that there will never be a single answer.

References

Altschuler, J., Black, D., Trompeter, R. *et al.* (1991). Adolescents in end-stage renal failure: a pilot study of family factors in compliance and treatment considerations. *Family Systems Medicine*, 9, 229–47.

Becker, M.H. (ed.) (1974). *The health belief model and personal health behavior.* Charles B. Slack, Thorofare, NJ.

Becker, M.H. and Maiman, L.A. (1980). Strategies for enhancing patient compliance. *Journal of Community Health*, 6, 113–35.

Bobrow, E.S., AvEuskin, T.W., and Siller, J. (1985). Mother–daughter interaction and adherence to diabetes regimens. *Diabetes Care*, 8, 145–56.

Close, H., Davies, A.G., Price, D.A., and Goodyer, I.M. (1986). Emotional difficulties in diabetes mellitus. *Archives of Disease in Childhood*, 61, 337–40.

Dunbar, J. and Stunkard, A.J. (1979). Adherence to diet and drug regimen. In *Nutrition, lipids and coronary heart disease*, (ed. R. Levy, R. Rifkind, B. Dennis, and N. Ernst). Raven Press, New York.

Eiser, C. (1993). *Growing up with a chronic disease*. Jessica Kingsley, London.

Fink, D., Malloy, M.J., Cohen, M., Greycloud, M.A., and Martin, F. (1969). Effective patient care in the pediatric ambulatory setting: a study of the acute care clinic. *Pediatrics*, 43, 927–35.

Fonagy, P., Moran, G.S., Lindsay, M.K.M., Kurtz, A.B., and Brown, R. (1987). Psychological adjustment and diabetic control. *Archives of Disease in Childhood*, 62, 1009–13.

Francis, V., Korsch, B.M., and Morris, M.J. (1969). Gaps in doctor–patient communication: patients' response to medical advice. *New England Journal of Medicine*, 280, 535–40.

Harkaway, J.E. and Madsen, W.C. (1989). A systematic approach to medical noncompliance: the case of chronic obesity. *Family Systems Medicine*, 7, 42–65.

Haynes, R.B., Taylor, D.W., and Sackett, D.L. (ed.) (1979). *Compliance in health care*. Johns Hopkins University Press, Baltimore.

La Greca, A.M. (1988) Adherence to prescribed medical regimens. In *Handbook of pediatric psychology*, (ed. D.K. Routh). The Guilford Press, New York.

La Greca, A.M. (1990). Issues in adherence with pediatric regimens. *Journal of Pediatric Psychology*, 15, 423–36.

Lansdown, R. and Walker, M. (1991). *Your child's development*. Frances Lincoln, London.

Madsen, W.C. (1992). Problematic treatment: interaction of patient, spouse and physician beliefs in medical noncompliance. *Family Systems Medicine*, 10, 365–83.

Mattar, M.E., Markello, J., and Jaffe, S.J. (1975). Pharmaceutic factors affecting pediatric compliance. *Pediatrics*, 55, 101–8.

Rissman, R. and Rissman, B.Z. (1987). Compliance. *Family Systems Medicine*, 5, 446–67.

14

Counselling

Attitudes to patients, adults as well as children, have changed enormously since the early years of the twentieth century. Then the physical examination and by extension the physical treatment of the patient was dominant: between 1905 and 1938 Cabot's manual on physical diagnosis made no reference to eliciting the patient's own history and even when it was included in other texts, for example in Stevens's medical diagnosis of 1910, it was given little space, being described significantly as 'an interrogation'. Beyond the disease, the patient was merely a passive receptacle—a good, bad, or indifferent historian, without an independent view. Two world wars and the rise of psychoanalysis changed all that. A 1946 *Lancet* article reminded doctors that allaying anxiety was of great value and by 1949 Hutchinson's 12th edition of clinical methods advocated that history taking should include the patient's mental attitudes to his life and work, ambitions, anxieties ... psychological make up ... hobbies and fears.' By 1976 the wheel had turned full circle. McLeod's (1976) *Clinical Examination* had 'The doctor's first task is to listen and to observe, not only to obtain information about the current problem but also to understand the patient as a person (Moynihan 1993).

Within a paediatric setting now we can see parents and patients as together forming a partnership with professional staff, not only at the time of diagnosis but throughout the course of treatment and, sometimes, beyond.

Definitions of counselling

When we write of partnerships, are we really talking about more than the recognition by doctors that patients have feelings? One of the difficulties in getting to grips with counselling in health care is that it is carried on, quite appropriately on many occasions, by nurses, play specialists, doctors, and others who are not themselves trained in this field. Indeed, although there is a recognized qualification, anyone may use the title counsellor, or psychotherapist for that matter, whether they have been trained or not.

To widen the debate even more one can invoke the notion that anyone who has contact with children or their families is likely to have some emotional effect on them, from the welcoming smile (or scowl) of the porter to the formal counselling of someone with an appropriate title.

Davis (1993) follows this line with his definition of counselling:

My definition is deliberately broad and refers to any situation in which there is mutual agreement that one person should interact with another in an attempt to help ... Defined in this way, counselling can refer to a wide range of situations, potentially encompassing the work of all health care professionals who have patient contact.

Noonan (1983) sees counselling as filling the gap between psychotherapy and friendship.

The British Association for Counselling (1984) have given a rather stricter definition:

People become engaged in counselling when a person, occupying regularly or temporarily the role of counsellor, offers and agrees explicitly to give time, attention and respect to another person or persons, who will temporarily be in the role of client. The task of counselling is to give the client an opportunity to explore, discover and clarify ways of living more resourcefully and towards greater well-being.

Although I would prefer to change the order of these three components to discover, explore, and clarify, the basic principle seems clear.

Neither the broad Davis (1993) approach nor the British Association for Counselling (1984) definition lead to an unequivocal cut-off point between counselling and psychotherapy. One way of looking at the two, while acknowledging that there are overlaps of technique, is to see psychotherapy as appropriate for chronic patterns of difficulty giving rise to dissatisfaction independent of any single event, whereas counselling is tied to a loss or incident (Farrell 1993). This is not perfect, for a single event can lead to a train of more general neuroses more properly dealt with in psychotherapy, while counselling can be appropriate for the general malaise that may accompany illness.

Davis (1993) sees the essential differences as lying in additional elements present in psychotherapy, including a more formal relationship, the explicit concern for psychological and social issues, a wider range of techniques, and more extensive training.

Needs for counselling

There is a continuum, from the least to the most needy. At one end is John A. He has come to hospital for the insertion of grommets, a procedure he understands. He lives nearby and the hospital is familiar both as a building and in terms of the staff. His mother will be with him and he will be with staff he knows already from previous visits. His last episode in hospital was a happy one and he has been looking forward to this one.

At the other end is John B and his family. They live 120 miles away from the city where the hospital is located, a city they rarely visit in normal times. Mr and Mrs B are farmers; but as they have very little help they cannot afford much time away. But John B has a lump which their general practitioner thinks may be malignant. John B has never been in hospital before, his mother is with him as often as she can be, but she is in a high state of anxiety.

The aims and objectives of counselling

The B family are examples of people thrown off course. Their predicament was summed up by Bawden (1974), in her novel, *George beneath a paper moon*:

The really unexpected happens so seldom that few of us know how to deal with it. We all move, for most of the time, in a small circle of known possibilities to which we have learned the responses. Outside this circle lies chaos, a dark land without guidelines.

Counselling cannot give guidelines but it can help the B family and others like them, find their own, establishing some order in the chaos into which they have been catapulted.

The specific objectives have been discussed by Hilton (*op. cit.*) in the context of counselling parents of chronically sick children; the list that follows is an adaptation of his proposals.

He begins by discussing the family's need to adapt to the new situation. For most they will find themselves bewildered, their old frames of reference about living no longer sufficient to meet the new demands. They will have to change the way they construe themselves, their child, disease, their partner, their other children, their daily routine, and possibly even their philosophy of life. Children, too, may need to change in all these areas.

Counselling can help, immediately and throughout the course of the child's illness, in the following ways.

1. By supporting families emotionally and socially.

2. By enhancing their self esteem, 'helping them feel good about themselves'.

3. By increasing their sense of feeling in control. (This applies to children as well as parents.)

4. By helping them to explore their situation so that they will be better able to understand and anticipate events.

5. By enabling parents and children to communicate with each other to maximize the child's psychological well-being.

6. By enabling them to develop coping strategies.

7. By enabling parents to find their own support systems.

8. By enabling families to communicate effectively with professionals.

9. By enabling them to make decisions for themselves.

Theories of counselling

No single theory is paramount, although one can argue that certain approaches may be more relevant than others. Davis (1993) writes from the standpoint of personal construct psychology, while Crompton (1992) touches on eight theories which can underpin this type of work. The important points are first that practitioners should have some theory to illuminate and guide what they do and, second, that they should avoid the twin pitfalls of rigidity and woolliness.

The art and craft of counselling

The next section will cover some points relevant to those who find themselves counselling almost despite themselves, nurses, doctors, play specialists, therapists, or whoever.

(There is, incidentally, much overlap between the skills involved in counselling and those techniques discussed in Chapter 5 on communicating with children.)

A starting point for helping is learning to know oneself, to be aware of one's own basic temperament, of weak and strong spots, of what may get one going in an irrational way, of topics that may be, for a number of reasons, sensitive. If there are areas of ourselves that we refuse to contemplate, we may not properly acknowledge them in others and then cannot be of help. This does not mean, of course, that helpers are perfect: as Egan (1982) has put it, 'Skilled helpers have their own human problems, but they do not retreat from them.' Neither is it argued that counsellors have to have a shared experience with their clients (or whatever they are called). Rather one has to be with another person, 'there where it hurts' (Tschudin 1991).

Most writers agree that there are three essential elements in the process: genuineness, warmth, and empathy. This may seem rather obvious, like saying clergymen are against sin, but the three can be unpacked a little to explain what they really mean.

The idea of genuineness can be illuminated by the term congruence or realness as Rogers (1980) often does. When our work self and our true self come together we can act effectively.

Genuineness involves giving the message that we accept and respect the other person, if possible, unconditionally. For some clients, for example those with low self-esteem, the very act of having been accepted in this way can be therapeutic. Warmth, incidentally, does not mean being effusive. The insincerity of the inept person who has learnt that one should give praise or compliments as a way of gaining influence over someone else is palpable and off-putting.

The unconditional nature of acceptance is not easy. We can say that we like the opening shots of a film but not its ending but when counselling we take on an acceptance of the whole person or, more accurately, we try to do this, for none of us is perfect.

Respect is related to accepting, giving the message that we believe in others' abilities to cope. We have also to get across the idea of trust: just as parents and children we meet will have varying degrees of trust in professionals, so they will have varying degrees of the sense in which they are trusted.

Linked to this is the respect one must have for others' perceptions. As is discussed in Chapters 8 and 9 when stress is considered, everything depends not on an event but on people's perceptions of that event and on their perception of their ability to cope with the demands it throws up. Here we may encounter, in various forms, one of the knottiest problems of all in this field. We may respect someone else's perceptions but at the same time believe that they will get in the way of a child's treatment.

Six year old Michael and his mother were both dying of AIDS. His withdrawn behaviour strongly suggested that he was aware that something was up and the ward staff wanted to allow him the chance to talk and to ask questions about his condition. But his mother forbade this, saying it was contrary to her culture to tell children anything about their illness.

It has been said that counselling is based on feelings. While I do not disagree with this, it should be added that feelings are necessary but not sufficient. It is true that part of the counselling process is experiencing and displaying empathy; we must, then, feel with and for the other person. However, this does not mean allowing our own feelings to spill over and distort our work. Empathy should not lead to the counsellor breaking down to the extent that he or she has to be consoled by the client.

And it is not difficult, especially for staff in a children's hospital who are themselves parents, to find oneself in a situation which rings bells in one's own life. We return to the need to know oneself, to understand one's feelings.

The power relationship

Although the formerly held view that doctor or nurse knows best is diminishing there is inevitably some inequality between staff member, parent, and child. Sometimes parents work to overcome this by behaving in an overbearing way; some read up the medical texts and have more specialized knowledge than those looking after their child. Yet if counselling is to be successful there has to be an implicit, and sometimes explicit, message of partnership, which is not the same as equality.

The process and content of counselling

There are a number of components. The process of counselling is simple, at least in theory. The exercise is essentially goal orientated: first the problem is defined, then there is an exploration of what a goal might be and then the counsellor and client work together to find ways of getting to that goal. A distinction should be made between counselling and problem solving: counselling is about helping a person with a problem, not about solving it for him or her.

Attending

An everyday experiment that psychology students sometimes try out when in company illustrates the power of attention. All you need do is start a conversation with someone and look attentively at that person during the conversation. Then, after a few minutes, shift your gaze. Very soon afterwards the other person will lose interest.

So, when communicating with a child or parent, it sounds simple; all you have to do is pay attention to the person you are working with. But paying attention involves far more than just looking. You are with this person in body, mind, and spirit, imparting the sense that your client is the only person that matters at that moment. Above all, if one is 'just listening', one must listen actively.

At the risk of sounding facetious one has to attend to the paying of attention. This includes sitting so that everyone is more or less at the same height, preferably with no desk or table getting in the way, making sure that your body is appropriately angled to face the other person. Body language conveys much: if you fold your arms across your body or lean away you will give messages that you are keeping your distance. At times, of course, you may want to do this.

At the same time the others' body language can be observed. Are they tensed up, leaning forward to hear what is being said, are they turning away, are they relaxed and open?

The tone of voice adopted by the other person can reveal much. With children, the mood demonstrated by the voice is usually obvious, less so with adults but still a source of information. What is often most helpful is to notice a change in tone from one session to the next.

Sometimes just attending can be therapeutic. A very distressed mother of an exceedingly sick child came to see me, obviously wary of psychologists, perhaps anxious lest I analysed her every word and interpreted her every thought. I sat, as still as I could, while she flooded me with her worries. At the end I explained that I would be happy to see her again but that she should decide about further work. She telephoned a couple of days later to say that she did want to return, adding, 'You didn't say much but you were very helpful.' During her full flow I had said nothing.

Related to this 'just listening' approach is the non-judgemental nature of counselling. This is harder than the textbooks often seem to imply for there are occasions when one has strong feelings about a statement or an attitude that has just been expressed. One way of tackling this is to ask oneself just how much help is really given to someone else when one comes down firmly to take a moral stance.

Exploration

As noted above, counselling has been defined as giving the client an opportunity to explore, discover, and clarify ways of living more satisfyingly and resourcefully.

Sometimes the task of establishing the main topic is, superficially at least, straightforward: I need help to cope with my husband having left; I can't face the thought of going to a new school and being teased about my face.

Even when the topic and the goal are clear there will be a high degree of uncertainty about the personality and strengths of the client. At times like this I explain that we are going to do a jigsaw puzzle together. The picture is that of the client. I explain that I know quite a lot about jigsaws but only the client knows about him or her self, so we have to explore together to see what kind of picture we are dealing with and how the pieces fit together. From time to time we will see how two pieces come to join: we will have made a discovery.

So first comes the period when neither of us is quite sure how the picture is going to turn out, when we are exploring in a wide-ranging way to establish our topics and our goals. This requires an open mind on both sides, not always easy in a medical setting where parents in particular are accustomed to highly focused discussions, with doctors expected to make firm pronouncements. Permission to wander, within reason, is one of the first messages to get across. The mother of a child with eczema is used to talking about creams and wet wraps and itching; she may need permission to stray into thoughts about her own childhood and how her parenting skills were determined by her desire not to be like her own inadequate mother and how guilty she feels because she is not reaching the impossibly high standards she has set herself.

Once again, this is not as easy as it may sound, for no matter how much the counsellor may encourage exploration, clients may still worry that this will be time wasting, so programmed have they become to the rush of hospitals. Two explanations can help here. The first is to share the fact that neither of you, at this early stage, really understands just what is going to be the most helpful areas to talk and think about and so some exploration is essential. The other is to make clear from the outset how long each session is going to be.

Part of the exploration may go beyond events to the feelings associated with them. Parents of sick children seem to have an insatiable need to talk of the events and their feelings at the time of diagnosis; bereaved parents will repeat what happened when their child died 10, 20, 100 times. With each telling something new may be learnt or dealt with.

Listening and questioning

There may, at times, be no more to counselling than listening—but if you know how to ask questions you will listen all the better. Tschudin (1991) uses a framework, based on several models, which involves asking the client four questions.

The first question is 'what is happening?' (What is being said or not said? What is going on?)

The second is to ask about meanings, what significance the topics of discussion have, what patterns they may demonstrate.

Third comes, 'what is your goal? What is the long-term aim and what is the aim of what is happening right now?'

Finally there is, 'what might you do to achieve the goal?'

These four keep the focus on the client; they make him or her work, they are open questions (see below and Chapter 5 for a discussion of open and closed questions), and they can be relevant to an evaluation of the process.

Tomlinson, quoted in Tschudin (1991), sees questions as having six functions:

(1) gathering information;

(2) encouraging conversation;

(3) identifying problems and difficulties;

(4) focusing attention on specific issues or topics;

(5) expressing interest in others;

(6) discovering attitudes and opinions of others.

Hargie *et al.* (1981) see questions falling into nine types.

1. Recall involves the recollection of information, most commonly used at the beginning of sessions.

2. Process questions ask for opinions and judgements; they encourage a deeper exploration of a topic.

3. Closed questions are those to which there is usually only one answer or if there are more they can be expressed simply. 'Did you go out yesterday?' 'Yes.'

4. Open questions leave the respondent free to answer broadly, indeed, they encourage this response. 'What did you do when you went out yesterday?'

5. Affective questions encourage people to explore feelings and attitudes.

6. Leading questions guide the respondent to an answer. Compare 'How did you feel about that?' with 'Didn't you feel terrible then?'

7. Probing questions encourage the expansion or exploration of something just mentioned. They often take the form of asking for more information.

8. Rhetorical questions do not expect an answer and are often supportive, 'What parent would say anything different?'

9. Multiple questions can be confusing: 'Did sister explain what the surgeon is going to do tomorrow? How do you feel about that? How do you feel now?'

Reflecting back

Reflecting back to the client can involve two forms of response. The first reflects back to the client what has just been said.

I feel terrible today.

That's tough, really awful?

The second reflects back what is thought to be implied in the client's statement.

I am not going to take that exam.

If you did take it and pass, you would have to go away to university, wouldn't you?

Clarification

Once the initial stage of exploring is under way comes the process of clarifying, although these two go on, one after the other, all the time.

Clarifying can involve deciding on what the problem really is or helping the client make sense of what has been produced. The problem for the girl who was discussing whether she wanted to take her exam was nothing to do with her ability, it turned out to be related to the sense of conflict she felt: if she failed she would have let her mother down, if she passed she would have to go away from home and, in her eyes, desert her widowed, depressed mother.

One way of helping the clarification process is by summarizing a session, which can also help to give a sense of movement. I often summarize and make brief notes with the client still with me, explaining, truthfully, that this helps me to martial my thoughts.

Some people, especially when they are seeing a psychologist, are on their guard. They stick to facts, repeating what they have been told. One way to overcome this is to ask, pointing to one's head, 'Do you think that here or (pointing to one's stomach) in your guts?' This is especially helpful when working with parents of desperately sick children, who 'know' that their child has little hope but who still cling to the possibility of a miracle. By indicating that one can have thoughts in two places, two sets of thoughts in fact, one is giving them permission to be irrational and to explore this side.

Empathy

What on earth does this word really mean? Is it more or less synonymous with sympathy? If it is, then why bother with a new word? Is it part of psychobabble, the coining of a new word covering the paucity of thought behind it?

Actually, it is neither of these, for it really does have a meaning of its own. It refers to a dual capacity: the ability both to understand the feelings of another person and to communicate that understanding. In even simpler language, it involves getting inside someone else and letting that person know that you are there.

Several writers, for example Egan (1982), have commented on there being two levels of empathy. In the first there is a reflection of the words and ideas expressed to communicate a basic understanding; in the second there is less a reflection of words and immediate statements, more a reflections of feelings and underlying trends. This does not always involve words: one's facial expression, tone of voice, even one's own tears, can express empathy.

Usually, the primary level comes at the beginning of counselling, the secondary coming later. There are times, however, even when counselling is well advanced, when one might return to primary levels.

Goal setting

As noted above, an essential element of counselling is that it is goal directed. Goals may be specific and time limited, dealing with an impending operation, for example, or more general, like coping with bereavement. Common to many goals is the need to help the client, whether a child or an adult, towards a sense of direction.

Part of the process of finding a new sense of direction is the exploration of alternatives, with as clear a view as possible of the futures that might be expected, avoided, or hoped for. This does not mean that one helps others to erect grandiose new ways of life, nor even that one tries to look very far into the future. One of the first topics I raise with parents and sometimes with children, is how far ahead they can think. A simple rule of thumb is that the greater the problem the shorter the period, so sometimes parents will say that they cannot think beyond the next week or in extreme cases, beyond the next day or the next 2 or 3 hours. We then have a clear time frame within which to set our goals.

Having established that, one then moves to setting the goal itself, as precisely as possible, in a way that will enable everyone concerned to know that the aim has been achieved. There is all the difference in the world between saying, 'I will not eat so much' and 'I will lose 2 pounds a week for the next 3 months.'

Challenging

Challenging another person is one of the trickiest tasks. It is, at times, essential to achieve movement; it is, at times, a destroyer of relationships. By definition anyone likely to benefit from counselling will probably have got stuck somewhere, somehow. He or she will need to be challenged in order to face up to the need to make other choices, other that is, than staying in the same place.

There are a number of ways in which this essential part of the process can be made more effective. One is to start by building on people's strengths. So often there is a litany of complaint or self-pity, a declaration of inadequacy that at times may seem almost wilful in its comprehensiveness. One teenage client, who had spent hours complaining that no-one ever listened to what he wanted and how he had been pushed around all his life, was challenged when I pointed out that his facial expression affected the way I felt: when he looked depressed I felt miserable. This came as a revelation to him and we went on to explore other ways in which he could influence people.

A second is to help the client do the challenging. One group of bereaved parents had been going round in circles for weeks, almost wallowing in their grief. The topic of why they were meeting came up and one mother said, to the group as a whole, 'We've got to let our children go.' That became a challenging goal for the rest of the sessions.

In all this it is essential to be aware of how central a self-defining idea is to the client. Personal construct psychology puts forward the view that we all have core role constructs, that is notions of ourselves that are central to our definition of self. The closer one gets to the core, the harder it is to accept change, for to challenge a core construct is to challenge one's essential being. So we start with peripheral notions. Mary Z may be only mildly fussed about being accused of poor timekeeping; Mary X may see this accusation as an attack on her essential reliability as a person.

One effective way of challenging, once confidence in the counselling relationship has been established, is to ask the client to do the criticizing as though from the standpoint of another person. I tried this with a father who had denied that he had any problems, personal or financial. He produced three statements about himself as though coming from workmates and then, without my needing to say anything, commented on how they were all negative. This led, with very little help from me, to his admitting that he was depressed.

Counselling, like stress, is one of those often misused words which can be tossed into a conversation, lifebelt fashion, in an attempt to offer some straw of comfort. It can be exaggerated in its difficulty and its efficacy; it can be misunderstood so that it encompasses both a listening ear (and no more) and interpretative psychotherapy. If it is seen, as was mentioned earlier, as midway between psychotherapy and friendship, we will not go too far wrong.

References

Bawden, N. (1974). *George beneath a paper moon*. Allen Lane, London.

British Association for Counselling (1984). *Code of ethics*. British Association for Counselling, Rugby.

Crompton, M. (1992). *Children and counselling*. Edward Arnold, London.

Davis, H. (1993). *Counselling parents of children with chronic illness or disability*. British Psychological Society, Leicester.

Egan, G. (1982). *The skilled helper*. Wadsworth Publishing, Wadsworth, CA.

Farrell, W. (1993). Differing approaches to training and practice in counselling. *Journal of the Royal Society of Medicine*, **86**, 431–0.

Hargie, O., Saunders, C., and Dickson, D. (1981). *Social skills in interpersonal communications*. Croom Helm, London.

Moynihan, C. (1993). A history of counselling. *Journal of the Royal Society of Medicine*, **86**, 421–423.

Noonan, E. (1983). *Counselling young people*. Methuen, London.

Rogers, C.R. (1980). *A way of being*. Houghton Miflin, Boston.

Tschudin, V. (1991). *Counselling skills for nurses*. Baillière Tindall, London.

15

Surgery

There are times when reading about children in hospital gives the impression that there is something wrong if they are not all enjoying every minute of their experience. In fact, some disquiet on some occasions is to be expected, indeed, it is to be welcomed as a natural reaction to inevitable stress. Surgery is one of those stresses when we expect anxiety but we should try to keep this in perspective: Freud (1917) postulated the need to distinguish between neurotic and objective anxiety. With children, too, we can try to disentangle the two.

Preparation for surgery

In 1985 the National Association for the Welfare of Children in Hospital (now named Action for Sick Children) published their *Policy paper 2*, a statement on the emotional needs of children undergoing surgery. This document has five points, based on the theory that the better the preparation the less anxious the child will be.

1. Children need the support of their parents on the day of the operation.

2. Parents and children need preparation for a stay in hospital and need to understand what is happening on the day of the operation.

3. Children should be able to be accompanied from the ward by a parent who would then remain with them until they are anaesthetized.

4. Hospital routines should be adapted to avoid unnecessary stress to children.

5. Children should be returned to the ward as soon as possible after the operation.

The first of these goes without saying—now; it was less evident even 10 years ago. Preparation is discussed in Chapter 7 and most if not all of what is said there applies to surgical patients.

Preparation can be in divided into two: information on what is going to happen and on how the patient is likely to feel, both just before and after the operation.

It is essential to explain what part of the child is to be cut and why. Sometimes this is easy: an operation on the spine to help the child stand straight for example, is easy to explain and to comprehend. Sometimes it is easy to explain but much harder to discuss the implications, as anyone who has had to prepare a child for an amputation will know. Sometimes it appears to be an easy task but turns out not to be so because children add their own details. A conversation between two toddlers in the Great Ormond Street playcentre went like this:

What are you in for?

I'm having my eyes fixed.

Do you know how they fix eyes in this hospital?

No.

First they cut your head off, then they fix your eyes, then they sew your head back on again.

It might be thought that the first child was deliberately teasing, but a well-known study by Vaughan (1957), looking at children's understanding of squint operations, reported any number of anxieties based on partial knowledge, an example being the boy who said afterwards that he was one of the lucky ones because he got his own eyes back again.

Against this is the account given in Alderson (1993) when a 10 year old girl was asked about 'having the tops of her legs made longer'. She replied to the interviewer, 'I suffer from achondroplasia and I am having my femurs lengthened.'

Sometimes the giving of information is difficult because the operation is not easy to portray in drawings or any other concrete way; much neurosurgery falls into this category.

Alongside the giving of specific information is the need to ensure that children understand the limits of what will be done. As mentioned in Chapter 7, one 6 year old girl, in for plastic surgery to her nose, asked her father if she would be the same person after the operation.

Information on the nuts and bolts of the operation is necessary but not sufficient. There is also the need to talk about the sequence of events on the day: the pre-med, if there is to be one, the period when children cannot eat or drink, the need, perhaps, to have one's hair shaved, the anaesthetic, and, what is called in some hospitals, the special sleep.

All sorts of fears can surround this sleep. It can be very frightening indeed for a child who has heard of an animal being 'put to sleep' to be told that this is going to happen in the anaesthetic room. If not properly explained it can lead to children desperately trying to stay awake for several nights before the operation itself, fearful that they will be cut while they sleep. The special nature of the sleep can be played up to extend to the children themselves, to make them feel special. Having a notice on the bed telling everyone that this child should not have anything to eat or drink is common; some hospitals give children a badge with the same message to emphasize how important they are.

Some hospitals have a system in which the child not only meets the anaesthetist before the day of the operation but also has an opportunity to visit the anaesthetic room and the recovery room beforehand, to ensure that both are familiar. One surgical ward allows children to dress up in green gowns, hats, and masks to ensure that the anaesthetic room garb will be familiar. As with so much preparation, if one can ensure that what is encountered is both familiar and reassuring the battle is won.

Equally important, more so in some cases, is preparing the child for how he or she will feel after the operation. In most cases it will be enough to say that there will probably be a feeling of nausea and possibly pain but more complex procedures can lead to children waking up to find their movements severely restricted. The most extreme example I have come across is the situation when a child wakes up unable to speak and unable to see, able to move only one hand. In such cases it helps enormously to spend a good deal of time in explaining why all this is being done in the way it is and then having a dummy run in which the child has eyes bandaged, arms and legs restrained, and so on, 2 or 3 days before it all happens. If children are likely to experience phantom limb pain this should be discussed and techniques for coping practised before the operation. Guided imagery, as mentioned in Chapter 9, has been most helpful at such times.

There has been some convincing experimental support for the value of pre-surgical preparation. In a classic study, Melamed and Siegel

(1975) showed a 16 minute film to children aged between 4 and 12 years. The film included 15 scenes showing various events that most children encounter when in for elective surgery, the child in the film showing some anxiety but also exemplifying coping behaviour. A control group was shown a film of similar length but with no hospital-related content. Both groups were then given a standard and quite thorough preparation on the procedure they were to undergo. The experimental group showed less fear before the operation and parents reported fewer behaviour problems afterwards.

The day of the operation

The National Association for the Welfare of Children in Hospital document also examines hospital routines, focusing on the need to reduce trauma for children. They should be starved only for the minimum time necessary for safety. Gowns should be attractive and possibly tried on in advance and if a child refuses to wear one then there should be permission to go to theatre in ordinary clothes, perhaps loose fitting nightwear. They should also be allowed to wear underclothes.

The actual day's routine depends on the practice of the hospital. In some, children are wheeled to the theatre on a hospital trolley, others allow parents to carry young children, while others wheel the child in his or her own bed. Some have decorated trollies—Thomas the Tank Engine or some such favourite character can be used.

There is generally little room for manoeuvre on the actual day although one area for choice may be the pre-med. So many children hate needles and are calmed at the thought of something given orally. Some anaesthetists prefer not to use a pre-med at all. Two, Schofield and White (1989) studied 151 children aged 1–14 years undergoing day stay general surgical procedures and found that diazepam and papaveretum resulted in sedation but, in a setting where parents were routinely present for the induction of the anaesthetic, no difference was found in the ease with which the children were anaesthetized.

Going to the anaesthetic room

Who goes to the anaesthetic room with the child is still a bone of contention in some places, although the policy of having a parent present is slowly gaining ground. A 1987 report noted that 98 per cent of parents went with their children in the Royal Manchester Children's Hospital (Day 1987). The National Association for the Welfare of Children in Hospital document referred to above is unequivocal in asserting that parents, or a familiar person, should go with children and stay with them until they are unconscious. Certainly there are good theoretical reasons for this: they are based on the same principles that govern practice over parents being with children in hospital at all.

The arguments against parents being present fall into three categories: one is that parents may themselves become extremely anxious at such a time and will then convey their emotions to the child and perhaps to the anaesthetist. As long ago as 1967, Schulman *et al.* looked at the induction of anaesthesia in 32 children, half of whom had their mother present. There was no report of mothers causing any difficulty during the procedure, along with some evidence that some but by no means all children were calmer while it was done. There was no difference in the post-operative behaviour. The Schofield and White (1989) study, mentioned above, found that 10 of the 141 parents were 'less than helpful' during the induction, five of them becoming distressed.

Another is that parents can bring an infection risk, although the majority of paediatric anaesthetists do not subscribe to this view (Glasper and Dewar 1987). Bush (1990), a consultant paediatric anaesthetist, states categorically that such fears are unjustified.

The third is simply that anaesthetic rooms are often cramped and one more person just gets in the way. One technique to overcome this is for parents and maybe children as well to make a pre-operation visit to rehearse their parts. In a busy hospital this suggestion will be given a rough ride by some theatre staff but it is worth considering.

If the anaesthetist is adamant about parents not staying with the child while the anaesthetic takes effect it is essential to plan the parting since the worst possible course is for the child to be tugged from the parent's arms. One approach is for the parent to try to settle the child, possibly just after the pre-med has taken effect and then to leave.

There is one further point to consider: parents should not be pressurized into going to the anaesthetic room if they are likely to feel uncomfortable. Turner (1989) pointed to the need to prepare parents for the experience. By the same token, an anaesthetist who has been forced to accept parents may function less well than normally.

Ideally children return, once the operation is over, to their familiar ward as soon as possible; if it is thought that they may have to be transferred to another immediately post-operation then they should have a chance to visit the new environment and meet the staff. There is much to be said for the parent being present when the child wakes up. If the same parent was there during the anaesthetic it will then seem to the child that the parent never left. On the other hand, the physical arrangement of some hospitals means that it is not always desirable to have parents in the recovery room so this, like so much, is a matter for negotiation.

Play and surgery

Play centred around an operation is now commonplace on paediatric wards. Children can work through anticipatory anxiety by operating on their teddies, their dolls, even on each other. Equally, if not more important, is the value of playing through the experience afterwards. An understanding of the normal manifestations of post-traumatic stress disorder leads to the expectation that children may want to play out or draw their experience over and over again.

What happens in practice

A 1982 multicentre study, 'Anaesthetists and Children in Hospital' (unpublished), although now rather old, is illuminating. It was carried out by William Hain, an anaesthetist, in 11 centres (two in Canada, three in Scandinavia, two in Sicily, and four in Switzerland). His main finding was a very wide variation in practice, the second being a great uncertainty in the public at large in all countries visited about the duties, role, and background of anaesthetic practice.

His conclusion was that much depends on the enthusiasm of the anaesthetists. In some centres they are closely involved in preparation, even visiting schools in Sweden, Canada, and sometimes in Switzerland. In all but one centre the surgeon spoke to the parents before the operation, the exception was one where, it was reported, the parents themselves did not want the subject discussed. In all but two an anaesthetist visited as well.

Several hospitals had open days for children from the local community and approximately half offered pre-admission tours for patients scheduled for surgery, although only one dwelt at length on what happens during anaesthesia. The most elaborate tours were in Canada and Switzerland. In one hospital in Canada the tour included a tape slide lecture given by a theatre nurse, during which blood pressure cuffs were tried on all children and they were all given presents of Smiley badge electrodes and operating room masks and hats. Children were encouraged to ask questions and then visited an operating theatre nearby where equipment, including that related to anaesthesia, was demonstrated. The questions most often asked in all centres related to 'going to sleep'. A tea party with more badge presents concluded the tour. It was noted that fewer than one-third of those children invited actually attended this tour. There was a similar scheme for in-patients.

Two hospitals had albums of photographs to show children what happened *en route* to the operation but only half had any play staff.

In contrast to the attempts at careful preparation noted so often, one hospital frequently told children who were coming in for an injection, an ECG, and an X-ray that they were 'only going to have a photo taken'.

There was as much variation in the pre-med as anything else. In five centres the traditional narcotic/anticholinergic combination was relied upon, oral benzodiazepine was used in five, while one gave a narcotic, a phenothiazine, and an anticholinergic drug intramuscularly together with a rectally administered barbiturate after an intravenous infusion had been established. In one centre one anaesthetist did not always prescribe anything at all.

The ideal period for pre-operative starvation was also diverse, as indicated in Table 15.1.

Given the discomfort and possible hypoglycaemia associated with starvation in some children the author concluded that it appears that many anaesthetists could relax their rules while still practising safely.

At all hospitals parents were encouraged to be present while the children were given their pre-med and at four they stayed during the induction of the anaesthesia as well.

Table 15.1 Pre-operative starvation periods (in hours) in 11 hospitals

	After solids	After clear fluid
Babies	Average 5.2 Range 3–8	Average 4.0 Range 2–6
Infants and older children	Average 7.4 Range 4–12	Average 5 Range 3–8

From W.R. Hain (unpublished).

In three hospitals children were asked whether they preferred to be anaesthetized intravenously or by mask. In contrast, one had a firm rule that children with a body weight of less than 10 kg routinely had inhalation and those over 10 kg were given an injection. Still another variant was found in the hospital which used the age of 5 years as a threshold between the two techniques and two used only intravenous methods.

There were also wide differences in the children's recovery experience. Five hospitals had no particular area for this, while others had recovery rooms specially staffed. In Canada parents were excluded from the recovery area, while in Scandinavia they were encouraged to be there. There was no evidence that when they were present they were anything but helpful.

Post-operative visits were made to patients regularly in four hospitals, although it was not clear from the report that these interviews led to changes in practice.

The long-term effects of surgery

The follow-up study by Douglas (1975), discussed in Chapter 2, reported that children who had undergone surgery appeared to have fewer psychological ill effects than those who had been admitted to medical wards. This could have been because it is relatively easier to explain surgery in concrete terms than it is to talk about many medical conditions. There is, however, a small but significant body of evidence to suggest that the effects of neonatal surgery should not be ignored.

There is some evidence that neonates may grow up to be less competent, more active, and more impulsive than those who have not had the experience of surgery. Although the studies have been few, the fact that they come from such different cultures, Japan and England, gives some support to their findings.

Kato *et al.* (1993) from Akita, Japan and Ludman *et al.* (1993) from London both found that there appeared to be an association between the number of operations a young child experiences and cognitive development, particularly subsequent verbal skills. Kato *et al.* (1993) speculated on the number of stresses related to operations as such (there was, intriguingly, no correlation between the number of hospitalizations and IQ) while Ludman *et al.* (1993), who had studied children undergoing major surgery, felt that their results established the need for a much larger scale study to tease out the many variables that are undoubtedly operating. J. Stevenson (personal communication), from the London University Institute of Child Health, has looked at the possible effects of inadequate anaesthesia having been given to neonates, dating from the days when it was imagined that they felt little or no pain. He has postulated that there may have been a biological response to the pain of surgery leading to a modest effect on subsequent behaviour, notably impulsivity and activity levels. These effects are likely to be very much less in children who have been operated on recently since the use of anaesthesia is now more sophisticated than it was even 10 years ago.

See also Chapter 9 on pain.

References

Alderson, P. (1993). *Children's consent to surgery.* Open University Press, Buckingham.

Bush, G. (1990). Allaying the fear factor. *Supplement to Nursing Standard*, **4**, 10.

Day, A. (1987). Can mummy come too? *Nursing Times*, **83**, 51–2.

Douglas, J.W.B. (1975). Early hospital admissions and later disturbances of behaviour and learning. *Developmental Medicine and Child Neurology*, **17**, 456–80.

Freud, S. (1917). *Introductory lectures in psychoanalysis.* Hogarth Press, London.

Glasper, A. and Dewar, A. (1987). Help or hazard. *Nursing Times*, **83**, 53–4.

Hain, W. (1982). *Anaesthetists and children in hospital.* Unpublished report to the National Association for the Welfare of Children in Hospital, London.

Kato, T., Kanto, K., Yoshino, H. *et al.* (1993). Mental and intellectual development of neonatal surgical children in a long-term follow-up. *Journal of Pediatric Surgery*, **28**, 123–9.

Ludman, L., Spitz, L., and Lansdown, R. (1993). Intellectual development at 3 years of age of children who underwent major neonatal surgery. *Journal of Pediatric Surgery*, **28**, 130–34.

Melamed, B.G. and Siegel, L.J. (1975). Reduction of anxiety in children facing hospitalization and surgery by use of filmed modeling. *Journal of Consulting and Clinical Psychology*, **43**, 511–21.

Schofield, N. McC. and White, J.B. (1989). Interrelations among children, parents, premedication and anaesthetists in paediatric day stay surgery. *British Medical Journal*, **299**, 1371–5.

Schulman, J.L., Foley, J.M., Vernon, D.T.A., and Allan, D. (1967). A study of the effect of the mother's presence during anaesthesia induction. *Pediatrics*, **39**, 111–14.

Turner, L. (1989). Creating the right atmosphere. *Nursing Times*, **85**, 34–5.

Vaughan, G.F. (1957). Children in hospital. *Lancet*, **272** (2), 1117–20.

16

Accident and emergency departments

Most children will have been to an accident and emergency department at least once before the age of 5 years. Twenty-five per cent of children will visit an accident and emergency department in any one year, a total of some 205 million in England and Wales. In one study of 399 consecutive emergency admissions to a children's hopsital in Nottingham, Wynne and Hull (1977) found that 61 per cent had been brought straight to the hospital either by their parents or by an ambulance after a 999 call.

Trauma is a frequent cause of attendance in hospitals; it is now also the most common cause of death in children over 1 year of age in Britain. The types of trauma vary with age: in the very young, choking, drowning, thermal injuries, falls, and child abuse are the commoner causes, while in the school-aged child road traffic accidents take over.

When a child attends an accident and emergency department the panoply of careful preparation mentioned in earlier chapters goes by the board; even the word emergency carries a considerable charge. Here are children who, unless they have been prepared in a general way at school or at home, will find themselves in a medical setting out of the blue. When one considers that this is likely to be their first personal encounter with a hospital and that experiences then can have a lasting influence on subsequent coping, there is all the more reason, then, to consider psychosocial factors.

Given the impossibility of preparing most people for admission to an accident and emergency unit, one early step to help everyone is to give newly arrived patients and whoever is with them some idea of what is going to happen in sequence. Figure 16.1 contains the major steps and can be used in some variation or other in a number of ways. Just putting the diagram prominently on a wall, with an explanation, is helpful.

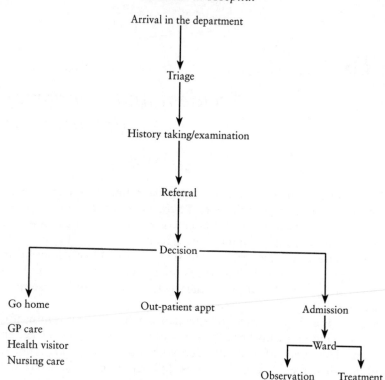

Fig. 16.1   The process at an accident and emergency department.

Triage can be explained as the assessment of a child which ranks patients in order of need. It aims to identify needs that require immediate attention. The age of the child is taken into account; younger ones will be more likely to have higher priority and the process may occur several times in the emergency department.

Parents of children who have had an accident present enormous difficulties in their own right. Even if no adults were clearly to blame, parents are likely to feel guilty as well as anxious. This guilt may manifest itself in various ways, one of which is anger which comes out as aggression towards anyone around, including the accident and emergency staff. It is extraordinarily difficult to develop rapport with this group, at least in the first phase of the encounter, and it is best to focus right away on pain relief, with a conscious effort to calm the adults with a display of efficiency and confidence. (Sometimes easier said than done.)

A second group of parents are those whose children have an acute illness which is thought by a general practitioner to be serious enough to be considered as a possibility for being an in-patient. Just being sent to an 'emergency department' can engender levels of anxiety that may stretch into the realms of 'what if my child is going to be seriously ill and might even die?'

Third come the so-called 'inappropriate admissions', children who would normally be expected to go to a general practitioner. Sometimes parents feel that their child is too ill to go to the general practitioner; sometimes the local hospital is more accessible that a general practitioner's surgery, or more friendly. In some countries there may not be a general practitioner to go to. This disparate group needs careful handling and it is unwise to generalize about them.

A fourth group, which may overlap with the first three, are those who have had little previous experience of hospitals, who may perceive any illness serious enough to warrant going to hospital as being the first page of a death sentence. Parents from overseas may fall into this category: having little to go on except their previous experiences, they may associate symptoms such as a cough, high fever, or diarrhoea with probable death.

Fifth are those who attend with children who have acute episodes of pain or illness that regularly require treatment and/or hospitalization; children with sickle cell disease are an example. These parents become worn down by repeated episodes and can become pushy, difficult, and aggressive because of their repeated distress. They are especially hard for junior staff, new to the unit, as yet unfamiliar with the range of treatment and approaches that have to be explored.

Difficult though these situations are (and it may help to see the problems as to do with situations rather than with individuals) there are steps that the staff can take.

The principles are no different from those that pertain for a planned admission, one of the most important being the need to help children and parents feel as comfortable and secure as they can in strange surroundings. As mentioned in Chapter 5, one parent reflected to me on what he most appreciated when he first met medical staff. It was not kindness or sympathy or even politeness: it was what he described as 'brisk optimism' by which I took it that he had welcomed the implicit message that the hospital staff knew what they were doing and were going to get on with the job.

But briskness in not enough, there has to be a recognition of the human being in the parent and the child.

At times like this children's greatest need is to be with a parent, but children often come in without any family members; accidents and emergencies cannot be arranged to order. When this happens it is a help to have one nurse remain consistently with the child to provide support until parents or some other familiar person arrives.

While waiting for a parent, staff can do much to try to calm a very young child, by talking softly and by offering opportunities for self-comforting activities like the sucking of a favourite finger. Children may have to wait quite a long time before being seen and Klinzing and Klinzing (1977) made the point that it helps if a staff member comes periodically to reassure everyone that they have not been forgotten. The same authors argued for soundproofed treatment rooms where children could be shielded from the more frightening sights and sounds of critically injured patients.

The realization that babies can feel pain is now common and it is of the utmost importance to watch for pain behaviours in the very young (see Chapter 9).

Even when they are with their parents, toddlers are particularly difficult. They are just beginning to develop a sense of autonomy; the well-known 'me do it' period is upon them. When they are whisked off to hospital they find that all this newly won power is taken from them. Just to add to the confusion they may regress in the face of trauma and behave in a much younger fashion than their years would predict.

Toddlers are likely, come what may, to show stranger anxiety and thoughtful early approaches can pay off. One technique is not to approach the child directly at all but to talk only to the accompanying adult, bringing the child into the conversation gradually. This gives the child a chance to sum up this strange adult and to come to terms with the voice, the manner, the appearance. A sense of calmness and lack of hurry is of enormous importance in these first few minutes.

Children who are extremely upset often respond to a toy, preferably one that moves in some way. An out-patient nurse I worked with for several years could win over almost any frightened child with a puppet that could take on various moods to suit the moment. A few minutes spent in talking and playing before attempting to examine a child can be of enormous value. One of the most elementary acts, elementary yet sadly often ignored, is to get down to a child's level. How often have we seen a frightened child surrounded by adults towering above? (It was even worse in the days when doctors wore white coats in hospital.) It does not take much to kneel down.

Although preparation cannot be undertaken in detail there can still be some warning before certain procedures. If an injection is to be given it does not take long to warn that it will hurt a little, only a moment or so to offer a choice of which arm it will be given in. It does not take long, either, to give some sort of reward, a drink, a special sticker, or badge, after it is all over. Even young children may benefit also from some explanation of why procedures are undertaken for they may otherwise construe them as a punishment for something they have done. Once such an explanation has been given it is as well to get on with the procedure as quickly as possible.

Older children, from 5 or 6 to about 12 years, will be able to talk about previous hospital experiences, valuable information especially if these were unpleasant. They should, if time allows, be encouraged to explore the equipment that will be used on them. The use of neutral language is helpful here. I once saw a child with a nasty splinter in his hand, calm if a little apprehensive, transformed into a wreck when someone said, bearing down with a sharp instrument, 'We'll soon dig that out.' Children can also be asked for imformation. As Phillips (1995) put it, 'It is important, particularly in the school age and teenage child, to recognise their need for self-determination both in imparting information about themselves and also in taking part in decisions about how treatment should proceed.'

The acknowledgement that children can express feelings is also of value. Much that is done to them will be painful or frightening or both and it is unrealistic to expect them to sit quiet as lambs. The old adage, 'shout as much as you like but try to keep still' is handy here.

Adolescents are sometimes branded as a breed apart, going through turmoil, creating havoc for themselves and everyone around them. This is a myth but trouble may arise if they feel that they are being treated as though they were children.

In some ways the needs of adolescents are, indeed, no different from those of anyone else. They benefit from having procedures explained before they are carried out, they need an opportunity to express their anger and anxiety, they need to exercise some control over what is happening to them.

But they are often emotionally vulnerable and need to feel that they are respected as people. One of the first rules, in any setting, not only in accident and emergency department, is to address them first, before talking to their parents or whoever has come with them. I usually ask the adolescent who he or she thinks is the best person to answer my questions. I do this with younger children as well but I try to make a point of it with the older ones.

One of the first tenets, not peculiar to an accident and emergency department by any means, is to call the child by name and not only by the name that is on the form but by the version of the name that the child prefers. A while ago I saw a teenage girl. She was not happy to be in hospital, even less happy to have to meet a psychologist. We began to get on a wavelength when I discovered that her preferred name was quite different from that in her notes.

Although there may be insufficient time to prepare children fully in an accident and emergency department, there is still the need to allow them, if they wish, to play out their experiences or just to talk them through. This will not generally be possible in the department itself but parents can be told of the importance of this 'debriefing' activity. Although it would be fanciful to say that all children attending an accident and emergency department suffer subsequently from post-traumatic stress disorder, some of the principles of treating that condition, the need to relive the experience in safe surroundings, for example, can be borne in mind.

References

Klinzing, D.R. and Klinzing, D.G. (1977). *The hospitalized child: communication techniques for health personnel*. Prentice-Hall, Englewood Cliffs, NJ.

Phillips, B. (1995). *Good practice for children in accident and emergency*. Paper presented at the Annual Conference of Action for Sick Children, City University, London, 1 April.

Wynne, J. and Hull, D. (1977). Why are children admitted to hospital? *British Medical Journal*, 2, 1140–2.

17

Adolescents

Adolescents, in the eyes of the World Health Organization at any rate, are people between the ages of 10 and 20 years (World Health Organization 1977). Their numbers in hospital have increased and are likely to increase further since so many more children with chronic and life-threatening illnesses are now surviving into their teens and beyond (Gortmaker 1985; Association for the Care of Children's Health 1988). The key question is whether they should have separate provisions. Despite a long history of talking, there has not always been a matching of action. The training of nurses reflects the vacuum: adult nurses are trained to care for adults, children's nurses are trained to care for children, considering their needs at different stages of development, but there is no special training in caring for adolescents.

When asked, many young people have made it clear that they would prefer not to be with or to be treated as babies and young children:

This is where I had my appendix out when I was 10 ... The same Snoopy mobile hangs from the ceiling ... The TV in the middle of the room is too loud. Fellow patients play with Lego and Alex in the bed next to me pees on the floor.

When the day nurses arrive they tell me I'm a good kid. I am 14, not a kid.

The play nurse comes and tells me there is a play room but seems relieved to see that I have got my Walkman.

The new nurse comes back and asks me if I have been to the toilet. She also feels moved to ask if I had a wash while I was in the bathroom. I truthfully answer yes. I want to ask her the same but I think she would find it impertinent.

Boredom takes on a new meaning ... I am beginning to feel thankful for the loud TV. (Steven 1992).

The idea of early lights out, Postman Pat videos and screaming kids did not appeal to me (a 17 year old).

I need my privacy, my own space, the right to do what I wanted. I worried about trivial things like whether I would have a room of my own or whether it would be a conventional ward with those useless curtains that make you feel continuously aware of the people next to you.

The reality was that he was admitted as an adolescent to young adult ward:

I was given my own room ... I had the freedom to go where I wanted when I wanted ... visiting hours ... were non existent ... there was a pool table in a separate room with TV, video and hi-fi. As well as this each room had a portable TV and sometimes a ghetto blaster. I soon realised that my fears were unfounded.

They can also recognize that they are not fully autonomous:

My only criticism was that I was given too much freedom with the IV drugs. The staff assumed I knew how to administer them myself as I had CF. They did not really talk to me about what I would have liked to happen to me or find out what I already knew. I guess I could have asked, but I felt awkward (a 16 year old).

(These last three quotations are from Tipping *et al.* (1993).)

Between them, these British quotes sum up much that can be said about the care of teenagers in hospital; they would like to be regarded as what they are, neither children nor adults. The anecdotal quotations can be supplemented by more large-scale work from America which gives a similar message (Rigg and Fisher 1971; Louis and Lovejoy 1975).

We should not be blinded by surveys and memorable quotes into imagining that all teenagers have similar views. I have known many who are quite happy to be with younger children and I have known some who long to be with adults. The best we can do is to look at the possibilities open to us in terms of provision.

One further general point: it is a myth that adolescence is inevitably a period of mood swings and rebellion; not all teenagers smoke, drink, swear, listen to loud music, and think about nothing but sex. 'As you grow up your age has a stereotype. I'm trying to escape from that stereotype' (Alderson 1993).

Adolescent units

A recommendation for separate adolescent provision is not new. It came from the Platt Report (Ministry of Health 1959), from the

British Paediatric Association (1985), and the World Health Organization (1986). The picture of how these proposals have been taken up varies.

In the United States the provision of distinct units for adolescents in children's hospitals doubled between 1981 and 1988; some 35 per cent of hospitals canvassed in a recent survey had such arrangements (Association for the Care of Children's Health 1988). In Australia there are few adolescent wards; 12.3 per cent of the hospitals discussed in a 1992 survey had one (Australian Association for the Welfare of Children in Hospital 1992). As noted above, there have been discussions on the need for more or less separate provision for young people in Britain for the past 30 years; nevertheless, over 60 per cent are nursed on adult wards (National Association for the Welfare of Children in Hospital 1990).

The debate often turns, mistakenly in my view, on the all or nothing idea of a separate ward or unit for adolescents. In specialist hospitals or in those general hospitals with specialist units, there is often an argument against separation: very sick patients need to be cared for by staff who know what they are about from a medical point of view. As medicine becomes increasingly sophisticated, so there is an absolute requirement that ward staff are able to meet the specialized demands of their patients. Yet it is possible, at no great cost, to adapt a section of a specialist ward to cater for older patients. This can even be achieved on a flexible basis, for example one plastic surgery ward known to me always tried to arrange that patients over the age of 14 years or so be admitted three or four at a time. Once in hospital, they were given beds or cubicles near each other and the ward social worker, herself quite young, held informal group discussions. In this way a portion of a ward was cleansed of Snoopies and Lego and could be given a more appropriate decor, easily removed when a new batch of youngsters came in.

Equally it is possible to provide a teenage area somewhere in a hospital, a room where young people can meet, listen to their music, talk, and just be. It is not suggested that such a room is unsupervised but the supervision can be unobtrusive and, if it be carried out by someone with counselling skills, there is an opportunity for informal support on a drop-in basis.

Ultimately, though, whatever the physical arrangements that may be made, the need, according to Gillies (1992), is for an alteration in attitude rather than a large increase in financial resources. Here we can pick up on some of the quotes given above: young people need, simply, to be treated as their developmental level requires. As well as the facilities discussed already, Gillies (1992) has pointed to nine issues to consider in detail.

The first is communication. At a mundane level is the need simply to communicate on an everyday basis and to do so in an appropriate way. In a children's ward the younger patients will often make overt demands on staff, leaving the often shy teenager to fend for him or herself. This can lead to a vicious circle of the teenager becoming silent and being labelled as difficult. Privacy is easily equated with having one's own space but again there is more to it than just that: a young girl patient in intensive care was greatly helped when it was realized that she felt infinitely more comfortable when she could wear a pair of knickers all day.

Independence is harder. It is all very well for a 15 year old to say he would like to come and go as he pleases just as he does at home but ward staff are responsible for ensuring that no harm comes to their patients and some control has to be exercised. The solution to this one relies, as so often, on careful negotiation. At a different level there can be some relaxing of rules relating to going about the ward: for example, some units forbid children entry to the ward kitchen, a rule that can be overlooked for the older patients.

Self-care, not just, 'did you wash behind your ears?' but one's medical care, can also be a matter of negotiation, establishing first what patients already do, what they are capable of, and what they would like to do. There are strict rules about medicine administration in hospital which must be adhered to but some care can be left to the patient.

The company of peers can sometimes be arranged by encouraging visiting from friends but if this is not possible then hospital youth clubs, guide or scout groups, or teenage workshops provide a focus for joint ventures which can lead to friendships.

The recognition of social needs may be particularly acute for this age group. Teenagers easily complain of boredom at the best of times and the relatively recent plague of video games will keep them quiet but is not a universal answer. Schoolwork helps in some cases, indeed, is essential for a number of teenagers approaching examinations, but most playrooms are not designed for this group. A hospital radio station can be an enormous help: the teenage disc jockey is not unknown. Sometimes patients find their own outlet. The boy who has been given an identification badge, with his photograph and the title 'honorary porter', mentioned on p. 98, is an example.

Legal issues present one of the trickiest aspects of adolescence in hospital, especially those involving consent to treatment. This is such a large topic that it is dealt with in a separate chapter.

Finally comes the need to prepare teenagers for transfer to adult care. Here the principles of preparation for anything new apply: give information, reassurance, and an opportunity to ask questions about the new setting.

References

Alderson, P. (1993). *Children's consent to surgery*. Open University Press, Buckingham.

Association for the Care of Children's Health (1988). *Directory of hospital psychosocial policies and programs*. Association for the Care of Children's Health, Washington DC.

Australian Association for the Welfare of Children in Hospital (1992). Westmead, N.S.W. *National survey report on psycho-social care of children (and families) in hospital*.

Gillies, M. (1992). Teenage traumas. *Nursing Times*, 88, 26–9.

Gortmaker, S. (1985). Demography of chronic childhood disease. In *Issues in the care of children with chronic illness*, (ed. N. Hobbs and J. Perrin). Jossey-Bass, San Francisco.

Louis, M. and Lovejoy, F. (1975). Adolescent attitudes in a general pediatric hospital: a survey of 87 inpatient admissions. *American Journal of Diseases of Children*, 129, 1046–9.

National Association for the Welfare of Children in Hospital (1990). *NAWCH update no 31*. Action for Sick Children, London.

Rigg, C. and Fisher, R. (1971). Is a separate adolescent ward worthwhile? *American Journal of Diseases of Children*, 122, 489–93.

Steven, D. (1992). Lump it or like it. *Nursing Times*, 88, 30.

Tipping, G., Schwarz, C., and Chapman, R. (1993). Teenagers' experiences. *Cascade*, 9, 5.

World Health Organization (1977). *Health needs of adolescents*. Expert Committee Technical Report Series 609. WHO, Geneva.

18

People who work in hospitals

Chaplains

Representatives of varying religions and denominations are frequently available to patients, parents, and staff on a part-time basis; larger hospitals employ some full time. Apart from regular services, they offer counselling and support to the children themselves and to anyone concerned with a sick child. In settings where there are a number of deaths they contribute to the terminal care service and, if numbers allow, are on call 24 hours a day.

Dieticians

A well-balanced diet is essential for health and well-being but there is more to being a dietician even than this may imply, for a number of conditions encountered in hospital require expert advice.

Dieticians work along with other disciplines to guide on the sort and quantity of food that is required and may engage in research on the subtler effects of food intake on behaviour and development. Their special skill is to translate scientific and medical decisions relating to food and health into terms which everyone can understand. Just two examples are the relationship between food and hyperactivity and the effects of iron deficiency on intelligence and behaviour.

Medical laboratory scientists

Medical laboratory investigation is one of the principal aids to medicine, assisting the medical staff in making decisions on the best form of treatment and helping them to monitor and evaluate the effectiveness of the treatment once it has begun.

The qualities needed of a good medical laboratory scientific officer (MLSO) are high standards of accuracy and observation and the ability to work in close collaboration with others in health care teams. Once qualified there are a number of areas of specialization.

1. Clinical chemistry is the investigation of blood and other biological materials by analytical chemical methods.

2. Haematology is the study of the morphology and pathophysiology of blood using sophisticated technology to count and size all types of cells.

3. Cellular pathology is the study of disease-related changes in the cells and tissues of the body.

4. Medical microbiology is the study of the microorganisms that cause diseases: bacteria, fungi, and parasites.

5. Immunology is the study of the immune system, which consists of cells, antibodies, and other factors in the body essential for good health.

6. Transfusion science involves the identification of individual blood groups and testing for compatibility of donors' blood with that of patients.

7. Histopathology is the study of patients' tissue removed during surgery or post-mortem in order to identify abnormalities such as cancer or heart disease.

8. Virology is concerned with various viruses, for example, HIV and infantile gastroenteritis.

Nurses

A shorthand way of describing a nurse's duties was put to me recently, by a nurse, as 'doctors cure; nurses care'. This seems to present both a gross oversimplification and an artificial distinction between roles. Nursing is changing in its remit in many ways, in many parts of the world. The overall pattern is towards greater responsibility, greater specialization, and a higher academic level of training. There is also a shift from a narrow interpretation of health care towards a wider view. As a Department of Health document puts it 'It is no longer enough to see the person as a collection of signs and symptoms; if we are to help individuals achieve lasting health, we need to understand their background, their relationship to society and the circumstances which affect health in their day-to-day environment.'

One recent development, at least in the US, Britain, and Canada, has been the establishment of specialist posts. These are usually linked with a particular condition, for example cardiology, and allow a unit to provide an outreach service so that families can be visited at home, especially useful for a pre-admission preparation. Because of the expertise that such nurses build up they can also act as a first-line support for families when the child is discharged and can be a bridge between the hospital and community services.

Similar specialization can be seen in examples like that of the psychiatric nurse who is able to play a role across wards, offering help whenever a child with a psychiatric condition is in.

Occupational therapists

Occupational therapists (OTs) work with people who have a physical or mental illness or handicap or a severe injury, helping them to overcome the effects of their disability and adjust to everyday living. This last point is of great importance for much of the work is related to day to day activities. In a paediatric setting there is a great deal of contact with parents and other carers as well.

The main areas of work include the following.

1. The analysis and training of daily living skills.

2. The design, making, and application of devices to assist or substitute for functional performance.

3. The analysis, selection, and use of equipment or devices for functional performance.

4. The selection of sensorimotor, cognitive, or psychosocial activities to develop or redevelop specific skills.

5. The use of games and craft activities to promote actions.

6. The adaptation of the physical environment to improve health and well-being.

OTs work in a variety of settings within a hospital. The most common unit is neurology but they can also be found in burns units, in those concerned with arthritis, diabetes, or many others.

Optometrists (ophthalmic opticians)

Optometrists carry out eye tests and prescribe and fit spectacles or contact lenses. They also give advice on visual problems and provide non-medical eye care.

The entry requirements are five GCSE passes in certain subjects with, normally, three subjects at A level. There is then a 3 year course of study leading to a university degree and a further year's clinical experience during which time the professional qualifying examination is taken before registration.

Orthoptists

Orthoptists are part of the professional eye care team. Their skill is in diagnosing and treating defects of vision and abnormalities of eye movements. Examples of problems are amblyopia, defective binocular vision, abnormal eye movements due to disease or injury, and double vision. Treatment techniques include occlusion, by a patch or by a cycloplegic drug, the use of prisms to control double vision, the use of lenses to change the amount of focusing necessary, and the use of exercises.

Research is playing an increasing part in their work.

Physiotherapists

In Britain, the Chartered Society of Physiotherapy has produced a leaflet entitled *Physiotherapy and me*. The following quotations are taken from that publication with kind permission.

Before someone becomes a physiotherapist ... they have to spend three to four years at a special college learning all about the body, how it works, and how to help when things go wrong. Some physios work with children and may do extra training to learn about children and the illnesses they get.

Physiotherapists treat people mainly through physical activities, that is exercise and movement.

Physios help children and babies to work at things that are difficult for them. This may be teaching children to balance and move better. It may be learning how to breathe and cough well if the child has a chest problem, like asthma or cystic fibrosis. They may help if you have got a broken leg or arm, if you have a really weak chest, weak muscles after an operation or painful joints.

Unlike doctors and nurses, physios won't give you medicine or give you injections. They help your body to heal itself. The physio may ask you to do special exercises to help you get better. The physio will explain and teach the exercises to you and your parents.

Physios will sometimes need to teach you how to use special equipment to help you move or breathe better, such as inhalers, crutches or walking frames.

Psychologists

In a number of countries there has been a great expansion in the interest in psychological matters in the past few years, leading to the employment of more and more clinical psychologists.

In some settings clinical psychologists are involved with out-patients who have behavioural problems or learning difficulties unrelated to any physical abnormality. However, the bulk of the work in children's hospitals can best be summed up by saying that it is primarily concerned with normal responses to abnormal situations. Thus, psychologists may find themselves helping a child who has developed a fear of needles or even of hospitals; they may support a child, parent, or whole family through the trauma of a child's operation or on a longer term basis throughout the child's illness. They may run groups for children, parents, or staff and may be concerned also with specific therapeutic interventions, for example, with children who have severe feeding problems. They may also help with the behavioural difficulties that accompany certain physical conditions, for example in units dealing with visual or auditory loss.

Neuropsychologists assess children with neurological dysfunction and may work also in the rehabilitation of such patients. Most other clinical psychologists working with children also spend some time in assessment but this is usually only a very small part of their work.

Increasingly, psychologists in Britain are becoming involved in the organization of hospitals. As clinicians are encouraged to take on more administrative duties so psychologists have come to do this, either as clinical directors or in an advisory capacity.

Radiographers

Therapeutic radiography involves the planning and delivery of ionizing radiation as treatment. Diagnostic radiography is the examination of patients, by means of X-rays, which are interpreted to aid in the identification of injury and disease.

Radiography equipment is becoming increasingly sophisticated and much of it is now computerized. New techniques such as MRI (magnetic resonance imaging) can give information about the body unthought of a decade ago.

Although it is a highly technical job, radiographers must be skilled in dealing with people for many children are frightened by the machinery and other aspects of the procedures that they have to undergo.

Social workers

Illness and hospital admission may make both child and parents more vulnerable and can thus interfere with the parents' ability to meet children's needs appropriately. The role of social workers as defined in Britain by the Central Council for Education and Training in Social Work is to try to help people cope with their personal, social, and environmental problems to live fuller, happier lives.

Often these needs are seen in financial terms, but there is almost always more to it than just that; social workers quite rightly bridle at being described as 'the money ladies'. (Apart from anything else, a proportion are male.)

Concerns about child care and child protection are frequently first identified when a child is in hospital and social workers *must* be involved when there is suspicion of abuse, which can include emotional, physical, or sexual abuse or induced illness (see Appendix 2 for guidelines and Chapter 12 for a discussion on induced illness). If there are grounds for action social workers will see that the child is appropriately protected. Much work in this and in other areas involves networking with local services, not always an easy task, for priorities in place A may be different from those in place B and tension, defensiveness, and even hostility between the two can emerge.

Other children for whom links with the local authority are required are those with complex illnesses or disabilities who have a high degree of dependency on a hospital and need long-term support.

Speech and language therapists

Speech and language therapists carry out the assessment, diagnosis, management, and treatment of communication disorders and feeding problems related to oral motor dysfunction. These include the voice, resonance, articulation, and receptive and expressive language. Thus, a therapist might be involved with a child with a cleft palate, helping first with feeding problems and then with speech, with a stammerer, with a child who has been severely injured in a road accident, with children who appear to be intellectually normal but whose ability to express themselves is limited, or those who for some reason are unable to comprehend the spoken word, although they may seem to understand gesture well enough. There is also much to be done for children who, for whatever reason, cannot learn to speak and who need an alternative or augmentative communication system, based perhaps on signs or a computer.

Treatment approaches include direct work with children but much work is done by parents and other carers under the therapist's supervision. Liaison with other professionals is an integral part of the work.

One of the best ways of understanding what therapists do is to examine their training in some detail. They study four core areas.

1. Psychology, including normal development from birth to old age, normal and abnormal developmental processes, and behaviour and psycholinguistics.

2. Phonetics and linguistics including the analysis and description of speech and language and its mechanisms, normal development of speech, voice, language, and fluency.

3. Anatomy and physiology including neuroanatomy, specialized anatomy of the organs subserving oral communication, and hearing.

4. Language pathology and therapeutics including the description, assessment, diagnosis, and treatment of disorders of communication.

Teachers

Teachers in hospitals can help provide a normal environment for children. Rather than asking 'What is wrong with this child?', they enquire what the children can do. Most children, in hospital for only a few days, will not necessarily welcome the opportunity to do some school-work, but those in for a long period often worry almost as much about missing school as they do about their illness.

....

19

Who cares for the carers?
Stress in hospital staff

Introduction

In his book on stress and health professionals, Bailey (1985) noted that 'Caring can damage your health.' While it is true that many of the studies carried out in this field are based on relatively small samples, providing an incomplete and possibly unrepresentative picture, a conservative conclusion from the information available is that working in hospitals can, indeed, lead to greater than average risks—but not everyone succumbs.

Definitions

There is considerable argument about the use of the word 'stress', as discussed in Chapter 8. The conclusion given there is that undue stress is the result of a mismatch between what a person perceives as the demands made on him or her and that person's perceived ability to meet those demands. In other words, no one breaks down from over-work: it is the worry about work that is so damaging.

There is little disagreement on two points: that a degree of stress is valuable, without it we would be bored out of our minds and that health care in any setting will inevitably bring stressful situations and demands. The key questions are related to why stress among hospital staff gets out of hand and whether there can be adequate ways of coping with it.

Burn-out

The concept of burn-out was born in the 1960s and has been flowering ever since. Graham Greene published his novel '*A burnt out case*' in 1961, describing a spiritually tormented, disillusioned, and despondent man, but it was the psychoanalyst Herbert Freudenberger who, in 1974, first defined the condition in the scientific literature. Originally applied to the caring professions, it is now sometimes widened in its application but the essential idea remains. Some people, beginning with a high level of idealism and energy, work in such a way that the job becomes a substitute for social life and they believe that they are indispensable. Eventually they reach a state of chronic emotional and physical depletion manifest in their becoming sullen, irritable, apathetic, and depressed, denigrating themselves and others.

The condition is often said to be found in people who are empathic, humane, sensitive, dedicated, idealistic, anxious, introverted, obsessional, and susceptible to identification with others.

Just as the word 'stress' has been criticized for being lacking in agreed meaning so has 'burn-out' (Farber 1983). In an attempt at increasing precision, Fischer (1983) sees the central feature as self-esteem. People who have been ground down by the stresses of their work-place to an extent that their self-esteem is significantly damaged should properly be called 'worn out'. The term 'burn-out' he reserves for those who cling tenaciously to a high sense of self-esteem, continuing in their tasks in martyr-like fashion with a desperation that goes beyond the reasonable.

Stress in the medical professions

The next two sections of this chapter deal with two groups of staff: doctors and nurses. This is partly because they make up such a significant proportion of hospital personnel and partly because most of the work on stress has been done on them. It is acknowledged that other staff have their problems and that all staff need support and understanding.

Doctors

Some data on the apparent effects of stress on doctors are frightening: in Scotland the rates of admission for alcohol dependence were found by Murray (1976) to be between two and seven times higher among doctors than among controls of similar status; a follow-up study of college students published in America in 1970 found that doctors were more likely than other professions to have poor marriages, to abuse alcohol, and to use sleeping pills and tranquillizers (Vaillant *et al.* 1970). In both the USA and Britain, doctors have a much higher risk of suicide than the general population; the risk in Britain was 72 per cent higher in the period 1979–1983, the latest available time for which figures are available (British Medical Association 1992).

The picture is not all bleak. An American survey published by Linn *et al.* (1985) found that their physician sample was as healthy or healthier than other population groups. They concluded, 'There is little in our data that suggests that our physician samples work longer hours, are more stressed, less satisfied or in poorer health than other professional groups.' So although there are no grounds for concluding that all doctors are walking wrecks, there is sufficient evidence to indicate that the profession is not without its problems.

Relatively little work has been reported on paediatricians as such. They seem less likely than others to commit suicide but at the same time have been shown to express lower job satisfaction than other doctors, at least in America (Mawardi 1979).

A source of particular difficulty, which applies to other professions as well, comes when they are treating children who are of the same age as their own. As one doctor put it to me, 'I feel that I am putting a needle into my own two year old.'

Nurses

Nurses fare little better than doctors. A recently published King's Fund monograph concluded, 'There is little doubt that occupational stress is a problem within the nursing profession. Rates of occupational mortality, wastage and absenteeism all indicate that the cost, both to the individual nurse and to the service, can be considerable' (Hingley *et al.* 1986).

Just as one should beware of generalizing about doctors, so it is imperative to avoid lumping together all nurses in all settings. It is important also to realize that the nursing profession has made considerable strides in recognizing its own emotional needs in the past few years and so some of the research published a decade ago may no longer be quite as relevant as it was. Certainly there has been a breaking down of some of the barriers that used to exist both between and within professions. Twenty years ago it was not always the done thing for a first year student nurse to speak to a second year without having been spoken to first; that has certainly changed.

The intensive care unit

Of all units in a hospital the intensive care wards should engender the greatest stress and produce the greatest trauma. Here are children who were well and happy on Saturday and dead on Monday, here are families who know that every child on the ward is, by definition, in a critical condition, here children are kept alive by machines which in some cases literally breathe for them.

The first thing that strikes many visitors to the intensive care unit (ICU) is not just the number of machines, the wires, and the pipes and tubes, it is the relative silence that greets a newcomer. The children running up and down the corridor, the crying babies, the theme music from yet another television soap are absent.

Activity abounds, however, with a constant checking of dials and screens and attention to bleeps from drips. Although it is now more than 20 years since Hay and Oken's (1972) summary, their words still ring true:

A stranger entering an ICU is at once bombarded with a massive array of sensory stimuli ... The atmosphere is not unlike that of the tension-charged strategic war bunker ... Unceasingly the ICU nurse must face ... affect-laden stimuli with all the distress and conflict that they engender ... But there is something uncanny about the picture the patients present. Many are neither alive nor dead.

With all this, it is not surprising that primary care providers working in paediatric and neonatal intensive care have been found to show higher rates of depression, psychopathology, and psychosomatic symptomatology than the general population, with extremely high rates of illness and burn-out (Marshall and Kasman 1980). There is also some evidence that the intensive care setting is more stressful than others in hospitals: two American studies have shown that in nursing there are higher rates of absenteeism, staff turnover, and drop outs among intensive care staff than is found on other units and, even more significant, those who leave tend to move out of nursing altogether rather than move to another ward (Walker 1982). Walker (1982) also noted that prolonged experience in the intensive care unit may result in behaviour changes in doctors such as preoccupation with non-intensive care unit activities and a reluctance to visit the unit, over-dependence on junior staff, inflexibility and resistance to change, opting out to other specialties, reduced output, poor problem solving, increased error, aggression, and diminished clinical judgement. The more cynical readers may feel that this applies to many consultants over the age of 50 years wherever they work.

Parents' views on their time on the ward can also be illuminating. Alderson (1990) sees the presence of student nurses as a critical factor; one unit she observed in depth was staffed only by trained staff and there the team was, in her words, more relaxed and confident. She goes on to discuss the ways in which an intensive care unit where the nurses are too busy and tense to talk freezes out the parents, one of whom seemed to think it was called an intensive care unit because there was so much evident tension.

On the other hand, there are some studies, summarized by Cataldo and Maldonado (*op. cit.*) which point out that on some units nurses are less stressed than their colleagues elsewhere, in these the staff have a high morale and often provide much mutual support. The most likely conclusion is that an intensive care unit is an area of heightened stress vulnerability but with careful management the emotional and physical pressures can be harnessed to provide support and job satisfaction.

The individual or the setting

Individual factors

Individual personalities have to be taken into account. A person who is temperamentally anxious will react in one way, while someone who is phlegmatic will respond in another. Many senior staff in hospitals are type A personalities: aggressive, competitive, tense, and moody workaholics. When everything is going well they can be productive, lively, valuable colleagues; when they feel that their grip on work is slipping they are anything but valuable. The concept of the individual stress threshold comes in here: everyone has an optimum level of stress; go far below it and one is bored, go far above it and one breaks down.

Vaillant *et al.* (1972) identified unstable childhood and adolescent adjustments as critical variables in physicians who showed emotional problems. But is there such a phenomenon as the doctor personality, a constellation of characteristics which leads people to medicine and in turn gives rise to increased vulnerability in the face of demands? In one remarkable random poll, Krakowski (1982) found that every one of the physicians polled declared that they were compulsive and all met at least three of the five criteria for such a label. The criteria include restricted ability to express warm and tender emotions, perfectionism, insistence that others submit to one's way of doing things, excessive devotion to work, and productivity to the exclusion of pleasure. Gabbard (1985) commented that the doctors' psychological make-up of doubt, guilt feelings, and an exaggerated sense of responsibility is reinforced in training. It is reinforced in practice as well; hospitals are often a world where working long hours, taking few if any breaks, is the norm. If one adds to that the pressure not only to see as many patients as possible but also to publish and to speak at conferences, we have a recipe for the compulsive personality to become supercompulsive.

The setting

Some argue that to concentrate only on individuals' processing and responses is to fail to see the wood for the trees, for it is really the system which is at fault. Maslach (1978) stated that 'The search for causes is better directed away from identifying the bad people and towards uncovering the characteristics of bad situations where many good people function.'

The British Medical Association (1991) is unequivocal in its condemnation of the system:

Almost three quarters of NHS expenditure is on staff, and yet the NHS has been called a terrible employer. Many staff are on very low rates of pay; training may be poor and drop out rates among, for instance, nurses, are high; the salary structure of most staff does not allow better pay for better performance; some groups work absurdly long hours in often poor conditions; career development is chaotic for some; sickness and accident rates are high; and occupational health services are often non existent.

The list of physical problems in any work setting is endless: excessive noise, cramped conditions, temperatures that are too high, a lack of light and air, and badly functioning or non-existent equipment are just a few that come to mind immediately.

Equally, if not more powerful in their effect, are human factors. Working with children who are extremely sick, who may die, is never going to be a picnic. But if one adds to this underlying factor the way some hospitals or units within hospitals are organized in rigid, dysfunctional hierarchies, where communication is bad and support for staff never thought of, where no one feels valued by peers or superiors, it is not surprising that one can find that this combination added to poor pay and physical conditions, can lead to high staff turnover.

If we add to all this the distress and anxiety caused by the recent changes in the National Health Service administration it is not difficult to see that problems are immense and widespread.

The system and the doctor

When looking for causes of strain, medical training is often invoked. It is both long and intense: a hospital consultant will have to spend at least 13 years first as a student and then a junior doctor before reaching independent status. One result of this constant pressure, it has been said, is that doctors do not have the time to grow up. Pfifferling (1983) commented that young doctors have no qualitative time to process their emerging identities, no time for exploration, for curiosity fulfilment, or personal growth.

The immensely long hours worked by many doctors, not only those in junior grades, is often put forward as another cause of strain. Working night after night with only a few hours' sleep, plus constant pressure when one is on duty, must impair judgement and reduce one's sense of competence. Not only is the professional life affected, the hours worked interfere with family and leisure life. Shaw, in his preface to '*The doctor's dilemma*,' (first published in 1911, Penguin edition first published in 1946) mused on why the impatient doctors do not become savage and unmanageable and the patient ones imbeciles. Perhaps, he thought, they do sometimes.

Long hours are not the only problem. Indeed, one American study in a children's hospital in Los Angeles (Werner and Korsch 1979) found that changing on-call rotas from every third to every fourth night did not improve staff morale. They argued that fatigue served to mask other sources of stress for the young doctor such as a new and overwhelming responsibility for patients, uncertainty about diagnosis and treatment, and lack of feedback on how well they were doing.

This duo of too much responsibility with too little support was illustrated in a conversation I had with a medical colleague some time ago. She had moved from one unit to another and was comparing the ways she had been trained in each. In the first she had been taught by the humiliation method: she was expected somehow to learn what she was supposed to do and her mistakes were made public. In the second she had spent the first week observing others in order to get a feel for the work to be done and the approach taken. She was then taught certain procedures, with an emphasis that there was always someone to ask if she needed help. Doctors have much to learn from other professions such as social work or clinical psychology in this area.

The structure of promotion in hospitals has been implicated as a further cause of stress for the junior staff. If one's career prospects depend entirely on a reference from one's immediate superior and if that superior is uncongenial there will be difficulties. As one surgeon put it, referring to his superior, 'You make one public enemy like this bastard and he can ruin your career ... It doesn't matter whether you're right or wrong or anything. You just have to take it' (Bosk 1979).

In the United States, there is an increase in malpractice suits leading to a huge rise in medical insurance and a rapid retreat from some specialties, notably obstetrics and gynaecology. When doctors are constantly looking over their shoulder, practising 'defensive medicine' by which every test under the sun is ordered in case someone should subsequently sue for their omission, the doctor–patient relationship is inevitably altered. No longer is the implicit message one in which a patient is seen as someone to be helped; now the patient is a potential adversary in court. Charles *et al.* (1985) point out that even doctors who have not been sued suffer from decreased self-confidence and indecision.

The system and the nurse

Although it was carried out in only one health authority, several years ago, the survey by Hingley *et al.* (1986) on nurse managers is a good starting point. They found first of all a high level of job satisfaction among the 515 staff responding. Since the staff had an average of between 15 and 20 years' experience it could be said that one would expect reasonable satisfaction in a group that had stayed in nursing that long. However, some 17 per cent expressed severe dissatisfaction; the survey highlighted eight sources of stress.

1. Work-load. There is too little time and, perhaps most importantly, too many conflicting priorities, made worse by staff shortages.

2. Relationships with superiors. This comes up time and time again in surveys: there is a lack of involvement in decision making, an absence of feedback from on high, and too little support.

3. Role conflicts and role ambiguity. These senior nurses felt that they too often had unreal expectations of themselves and of others.

4. Death. This can be seen as a shorthand term for the anxieties surrounding the care of desperately sick people; it is the deaths that

encapsulate the problems but there is so much suffering in other contexts.

5. Home–work conflicts. Many said that they could not switch off when they went home; a minority said that home demands inhibited their career advancement.

6. Career. There was a perception of low status and limited promotion prospects.

7. Interpersonal relationships. Difficulties were expressed with patients, families, and colleagues.

8. Physical resources. This can be expressed simply as not enough and what there is may often be of poor quality.

Although this survey was of experienced nurse managers, I have often heard similar points made by students and by those in other grades. (See the account of the study carried out in Great Ormond Street on p. 216) The lack of involvement in decision making can be particularly acute when a patient is in the terminal stage of an illness. So often there is a disagreement between nurse and doctor on how a patient should be managed. At its extreme this can centre around whether a child should be allowed to die or whether treatment should continue at all costs. Parents' opinions come into this, of course and, sometimes, children themselves have their say, but nursing staff who have become attached to a child feel deeply about such decisions and much resentment is caused if the decisions are made without acknowledging this.

The absence of feedback and support is a common complaint among all grades. (It is not that uncommon among other professions as well.) Role conflict and ambiguity among students is, in part, a function of staff shortages and, in part, a result of the system. As one student put it, 'One day I am treated like a child and then on another I am given too much responsibility.'

While there are grounds for supporting the British Medical Association's somewhat polemical view on the National Health Service, there is a danger of oversimplifying the topic. Indeed, the lure of oversimplification is one of the few points of agreement among commentators. Some have argued that the focus on organizational stress distracts and misleads those who are seeking to understand psychological disturbance in the work-place since it is practically useless as a foundation for treatment interventions (Duckworth 1985). Others have been more forthright and asserted that debates on stress and burn-out do no more than provide an excuse for the inadequate (Morrow 1981).

Responses to stress

Coping

First of all there is the need to acknowledge that there is a problem, which is not easy for professions such as medicine and nursing in which the practitioners spend most of their time assuming the role of the well-functioning person working with the sick.

Next comes the need to establish causes. One way to do this is to ask people straightforward questions, either about themselves or the setting in which they work. A second source of information is to interview all leavers: they are often more willing to say what they really think when they know that they have another job to go to.

Then comes the step of trying to do something about it. Here come a number of possibilities, two of which are rarely mentioned in books on stress management. The first is to accept that the person has simply chosen the wrong job. Working with sick children has its own demands not always found in other branches of medicine and care, and considering other fields may be the best solution.

The second is that the job may have altered around the person and that expecting personal change is to ask too much. Someone now approaching retirement will have been brought up in a world where the consultant's word was unquestioned; junior staff were there to be told what to do, nurses, parents, children, and administrators knew their place. In that world the idea of explaining one's decisions to a student social worker, listening to children, or determining one's clinical priorities at the behest of the finance department would have been unthinkable. Most of those old-style staff have now retired but there remains an element of the assumptions here and there.

The next decision is whether to try to change individuals or the system in which they work or both.

Changing individuals

Responses by individuals are usually discussed under two headings, the adaptive and the maladaptive. Under the second heading comes excessive smoking or drinking, denial of there being a problem, working even harder than usual, and emotional distancing of oneself from the work.

While no-one would advocate any of these as generally useful approaches, there are times when each, even the use of alcohol, might be seen as valuable in the very short-term. It is their habitual use which is damaging.

Some texts on stress management emphasize the role of individual factors in determining stress and in combatting it. Bond (1986) is a good example; her nine chapters deal with relaxation, meditation, assertiveness, and other personal elements, with encouragement to take exercise, to eat and drink sensibly, to relax, etc.

At a different level, staff can be helped to switch off when they get home and/or to seek support from family or friends if this is not available at work.

A third approach is to consider the need for scheduled time off, for enforced breaks (many staff work straight through the day with no break at all, tea and coffee are grabbed when there is a moment, and lunch is a sandwich while one continues working). The use of the sabbatical, a change not just a rest, has scarcely been considered outside universities.

One individual approach which is becoming increasingly used is the technique of time management and learning how to order one's work in terms of priorities. This is more applicable to senior staff, but it has its role for many others as well.

Another is goal setting, usually carried out within the framework of a regular appraisal of work. Appraisals are not, as they are sometimes perceived, disciplinary procedures; they exist in order to help individuals take stock of their present roles, their career plans, professional development, and their goals.

I have some sympathy with the view that all this is no more than putting a bandage round a finger when a blood transfusion is what is needed; changing individual behaviour may help, sometimes it may help a lot, but so often it is the system which needs attention. The two are not, of course, mutually incompatible and some of the proposals for systems discussed below involve individual action.

Changing the system

There are times when an institution as a whole adopts a coping mechanism which may not always be adaptive. One of the earliest pieces of work in studying this was carried out by Menzies (1960). She saw nursing, then, as organized in such a way as to maintain defences against anxiety by having rules about not getting involved with patients, by keeping 'professionally detached'. Many people working in the field today would argue that this was actually maladaptive in that it dehumanized contact and that it has already been changed. What has replaced it, one hopes, is professional attachment, that is an involvement with patients and their families which enables staff to have a human contact while retaining their integrity and not being overwhelmed by that contact. Whether the change has permeated to all staff everywhere is a moot point.

One of the first areas for consideration, that comes up time and time again, is to do with communication. If only Dr X had told nurse Y what she had discussed with the parents of that child, nurse Y would have known how to respond to the parents' emotions. If only the hospital administrators had told the head of department in advance that they would be taking away his rest room the department could have coped with the loss. Even better if they had explained why.

It is sometimes hard to decide whether poor communication is a cause or a symptom of a poor system but one key point is that it should be two way. It is admittedly very important to have an efficient, top-down, system to disseminate information; it is another to ensure that all the relevant people feel that they have a bottom-up opportunity to make their wishes felt in decision making. All it needs is effort and goodwill, on all sides.

A second area has a rather loose heading of 'support'. Cobb (1976) defined social support as that which leads to individuals 'believing that they are cared for and loved, esteemed and valued and that they participate in a network of communication and mutual obligation'.

Pines (1983) has looked at it under six headings.

1. Listening. We almost all need someone to listen to us, without making judgements, without necessarily giving advice.

2. Technical support. Work in all hospitals is becoming increasingly sophisticated, more high tech; one of the most common individual responses to stress surveys is a feeling of technical inadequacy, of not having been trained for the job. We need to be taught, not by the humiliation method but in a supportive framework.

3. Technical challenge. If we are not challenged we run the risk of stagnation. Taking on a new project, learning a new technique, is of as much value for the most experienced staff member as it is for the most junior.

4. Emotional support. An emotional supporter is one who is willing to be on our side even if he or she does not totally agree with what we are doing. Emotional support can and often does come from a team. When we are in a job where there are constant demands, especially when those demands tap skills that we may not feel we have, it is of enormous value to have colleagues working alongside

us, to share problems and also to help each other devise new approaches to those problems.

5. Emotional challenge. This is much more tricky than anything so far mentioned. It involves a questioning of effort and can easily slip into nagging. It is likely to come best, once again, in a team setting where the team members will question themselves as a group to see if they really are doing all they can in the situation.

6. Sharing social reality. This implies help from another person, whom one trusts, to test out the validity of what is being said or what is happening. It is often useful to share views on a new treatment technique, a new plan, with someone who will not necessarily follow blindly after the latest fad. There is some evidence that listening and emotional support are the most valued of these two.

The ward/unit support group

Support groups have been called upon as a means of preventing burnout or, to follow Fischer (1983), to prevent staff becoming worn out. They are one way of an organization formalizing the need for support. They are usually led by someone not directly connected with the working unit, ideally are held at the same time each week for a limited period so that everyone knows when they will end. They provide a safe place to ventilate feelings of anger, frustration, and depression and they allow a sharing of feelings and an opportunity for a group to try to seek alternative ways to present functioning in order to try to prevent problems arising again.

The psychosocial ward round

More and more children's hospitals and paediatric wards now have psychosocial meetings, attended by ward staff and the so-called psychosocial team. These have been mentioned earlier, (see Chapter 8) and can provide a focus for the discussion of problems experienced among the staff as well as the families. Often the opportunity to ventilate and discuss difficulties within a context in which psychological factors are at the forefront of people's minds can be sufficient but there may be a subsequent need to take matters further, either with specially set up meetings or in some other way. The study on the oncology ward mentioned below is an example of action that emerged from a psychosocial meeting.

From the individual to the system: reducing stress in the cancer ward

The second half of this heading is the title of an article in a nursing journal (Lansdown *et al.* 1990). The authors begin with an outline of some of the research into stress among nurses working with patients with a life-threatening illness, pointing out that recent work has suggested that staff are at risk for a number of reasons. They may have begun this work with high ideals but unrealistic expectations, they may find that the constant confrontation with death evokes past losses they have experienced themselves, the preoccupation with death that happens to so many workers in the field may mean that their ability to enjoy friendships outside the ward is impaired, and, perhaps most important of all, the frequency of deaths reinforces a sense of inadequacy (Vachon and Pakes 1984; Waters 1985; Wooley *et al.* 1989).

McDermott (1983) discussed the way in which a Canadian ward was organized in order to prevent undue stress. The first step is selective hiring, that is there should be care to fit round pegs to round holes. Next comes ongoing care, which includes senior staff being visible, communication being open, and an effort to identify individuals' talents. As far as possible there should be a choice of work assignments, with flexible work schedules. Professional growth is also emphasized.

Waters (1985) put forward ways of alleviating stress but there have been relatively few evaluated studies. The work reported by Lansdown *et al.* (1990) took place on the oncology/haematology ward in Great Ormond Street following discussions in the psychosocial meeting. A survey was carried out among all the staff to establish the perceived causes and extent of the stress experienced and to enquire into people's coping techniques.

A number of causes over which the staff could have little control were identified, a lack of space and insufficient resources being two. Others, it was felt, were open to change, such as the comments about lack of feedback from one's superiors and the sense of inadequacy in the face of the demands made.

There were 17 coping strategies mentioned, the most common of which was getting away for a break. Several people used more than one technique. The two that appeared to be the most effective were taking exercise and talking to colleagues, although a number of respondents mentioned support given at home. ('When I've had a really rough day I give my husband a three-line whip. We go out for a curry and he is not allowed to say a word while I bend his ear until I feel better.')

All the medical and nursing staff registered high levels of stress but the group appearing to be most vulnerable were the student nurses.

Following the survey, another sister was appointed to the ward, charged with paying attention to the points raised in the survey. Heed was given to communication, not just in meetings but in more informal settings. It may sound trite to say that it helps when staff talk to each other but it is true. It helps also when staff thank each other from time to time. Regular meetings were scheduled between senior nursing staff and consultants.

Formal support groups were rejected partly because previous experience and a reading of the literature had suggested that they are not without their drawbacks: there can be fears about confidentiality and they can be hijacked by one or two articulate members. (This is not to say that formal groups should never be considered, we have run a number for nurses which have been well received.) Instead, informal group support was offered to the students, particularly *ad hoc* groups held when there was a crisis.

A great deal of thought went into the orientation of new staff, getting away from the 'throw her in at the deep end' approach. This overt recognition of the fact that people should not be expected to know everything as soon as they walk on the ward was reinforced by senior staff being encouraged to seek help from others, thus acting as role models to those who might otherwise feel hesitant about revealing their ignorance.

An informal appraisal system was added to the formal one already in existence, in which each sister had four or five staff nurses who supervised the learners in a link system. Learners were encouraged to make constructive comments about the ward either face to face or through a suggestions box.

An attempt to counter the sense of professional inadequacy was made via an increase in formal and informal teaching; additional resources were put into the ward library and the tape and video collection and more opportunities than hitherto were given to staff to visit other hospitals to compare notes.

There was a focus on the appearance of the ward; pictures were bought and parts refurbished from ward funds and, finally, the staff social life was improved with a social committee being set up to organize parties and outings.

The evaluation was carried out in two ways. The first was a repeating of the original survey which indicated that while stress levels for the medical and senior nursing staff were much as before, those of the targeted group, the students, were substantially lower. The second was to look at sickness rates. Although the average length of absence was constant at 3.1 days, the number of sickness episodes fell from 5.1 per month to 3.1, despite an increase in nursing staff by five whole time equivalents, from 17.75 to 22.85.

References

Alderson, P. (1990). *Choosing for children*. Oxford University Press, Oxford.

Bailey, R. (1985). *Coping with stress in caring*. Blackwell, Oxford.

Bond, M. (1986). *Stress and self-awareness: a guide for nurses*. Heinemann, London.

Bosk, C.L. (1979). *Forgive and remember: managing medical failure*. Chicago University Press, Chicago.

British Medical Association (1991) *Leading for health: a BMA agenda for health*. BMA, London.

British Medical Association (1992). *Stress and the medical profession*. BMA Scientific Division, London.

Charles, S.C., Wilbert, J.R., and Franke, K.J. (1985). Sued and non-sued physicians self-reported reactions to malpractice litigation. *American Journal of Psychiatry*, **142**, 437–40.

Cobb, S. (1976). Social support as a moderator of life stress. *Psychosomatic Medicine*, **5**, 300–17.

Duckworth, D.H. (1985). Is the 'organizational stress' construct a red herring? A reply to Glowinkowski and Cooper. *Bulletin of the British Psychological Society*, **38**, 401–4.

Farber, B.A. (ed.) (1983). *Stress and burnout in the human service professions*. Pergamon Press, New York.

Fischer, H.J. (1983). A psychoanalytic view of burnout. In *Stress and burnout in the human service professions*, (ed. B.A. Farber). Pergamon Press, New York.

Freudenberger, H. (1974). Staff burn-out. *Journal of Social Issues*, **30**, 159–65.

Gabbard, G.O. (1985). The role of compulsiveness in the normal physician. *Journal of the American Medical Association*, **254**, 2926–9.

Hingley, P., Cooper, C.L., and Harris, P. (1986). *Stress in nurse managers*. King's Fund Centre, London.

Krakowski, A. (1982). Stress in the practice of medicine. II Stresses and strains. *Psychotherapy & Psychosomatics*, **38**, 11–23.

Lansdown, R., Pike, S., and Smith, M. (1990). Reducing stress in the cancer ward. *Nursing Times*, **86**, 34–8.

Lazarus, R. (1966). *Psychological stress and the coping process*. McGraw-Hill, New York.

Linn, L.S., Yager, J., Cope, D., and Leake, B. (1985). Health status, job satisfaction and life satisfaction among academic and clinical faculty. *Journal of the American Medical Association*, **254**, 2787–9.

McDermott, B. (1983). A preventative approach to staff stress. *Canadian Nurse*, **79**, 27–9.

Maslach, C. (1978). Job burnout: how people cope. *Public Welfare*, **36**, 56–8.

Mawardi, B.H. (1979). Satisfactions, dissatisfactions and causes of stress in medical practice. *Journal of the American Medical Association*, **241**, 1483–6.

Menzies, I. (1960). Institutional defence against anxiety. *Human Relations*, **13**, 95–121.

Morrow, L. (1981). The burnout of almost everyone. *Time*, 21 September 84.

Pfifferling, J.H. (1983). Coping with residency distress. *Resident & Staff Physician*, **29**, 105–11.

Pines, A. (1983). On burnout and the buffering effects of social support. In *Stress and burnout in the human service professions*, (ed. B.A. Farber). Pergamon Press, New York.

Vachon, M.L.S. and Pakes, E. (1984). Staff stress in the care of the critically ill and dying child. In *Childhood and death*, (ed. H. Wass and C.A. Corr). Hemisphere Publishing Corporation, New York.

Vaillant, G.E., Brighton, J.R., and McArthur, C. (1970). Physicians' use of mind altering drugs. *New England Journal of Medicine*, **282**, 365–70.

Vaillant, G.E., Sobowale, N.C., and McArthur, C. (1972). Some psychologic vulnerabilities of physicians. *New England Journal of Medicine*, **287**, 372–5.

Waters, A.L. (1985). Support for staff in a paediatric oncology unit. *Nursing*, **2**, 1275–7.

Werner, E.R. and Korsch, B.M. (1979). Professionalization during internship: attitudes, adaptation and interpersonal skills. In *Becoming a physician: development of attitudes in medicine*, (ed. E.C. Shapiro and L.M. Lowenstein). Ballinger Publishing Co., Cambridge, MA.

Wooley, H., Stein, A., Forrest, G. *et al.* (1989). Staff stress and job satisfaction at a children's hospice. *Archives of Disease in Childhood*, **64**, 114–18.

Further reading

R. Payne and Firth-Cozens, J. (ed.) (1987). *Stress in health professionals*. John Wiley, Chichester.

20

Ethical and legal issues

Although reams have been written on these topics, in the end discussions come down to one question: what should a person do? As Socrates put it, what we are talking about is how one should live. One way to start is to look at what we have been told to do.

Declarations

Extracts from the Hippocratic Oath (fourth century BC)

I swear by Apollo the physician, and Aesculapius and Health, and Allheal, and all the gods and goddesses, that, according to my ability and judgement, I will keep this Oath ... I will follow that system of regimen which, according to my ability and judgement, I consider for the benefit of my patients, and abstain from whatever is deleterious and mischievous ... Whatever, in connection with my professional practice, or not in connection with it, I see or hear, in the life of men, which ought not to be spoken abroad, I will not divulge, as reckoning that all such should be kept secret.

Extracts from the Declaration of Geneva (1968)

The health of my patient will be by my first consideration ... I will not permit considerations of religion, nationality, race, party politics or social standing to intervene between my duty and my patients ... I will maintain the utmost respect for human life.

Extract from the Declaration of Helsinki (1975)

In my research on human beings, each potential subject must be adequately informed of the aims, methods, anticipated benefits and potential hazards of the study and the discomfort it may entail. He or she should be informed that he or she is at liberty to abstain from participation and that he or she is free to withdraw his or her consent to participation at any time. The doctor should then obtain the subject's freely-given informed consent, preferably in writing.

Extract from the 1983 revision of the Declaration of Helsinki

When the research subject is a minor, permission from the responsible relative replaces that of the subject in accordance with national legislation. Whenever the minor child is in fact able to give consent, the minor's consent must be obtained in addition to the consent of the minor's legal guardian.

Moral rights and legal principles

Just as the emotional needs of children in hospital have increasingly been recognized, so there has been a corresponding rise in the awareness of their rights. This is not, of course, confined to children. There has been a similar shift for adults as well.

Rights are based on either moral or legal principles or both. Declarations on moral rights are often based on the thinking of the eighteenth-century philosopher Immanuel Kant, whose categorical imperative demands that a moral right is held to be universal: if it applies to one it applies to all. Being grounded in the good, a moral right should not be changed. They are not necessarily legally enforceable, although if enough public opinion is aroused on a topic, laws will be passed to make a moral issue a matter for the law as well.

A dilemma arises when there is conflict between two moral systems. The problem of the Jehovah's Witness who refuses to accept blood products is discussed below; it is a good example of a potential conflict between the moral system of the Jehovah's Witnesses and the hospital staff. As Faulder (1985) put it, 'We spend our time performing a balancing act, weighing alternatives and making decisions in relation to other people's rights as well as our own, in the full realisation that we cannot enjoy exclusive personal autonomy.'

Whether legal rights have to have any moral support, since the law is concerned only with what is right or wrong according to legal definitions, is a contentious matter. What is clear, however, is the fact that laws can and sometimes must be changed.

Patients' legal rights

The rights of patients in law are narrowly defined. A doctor can be sued for battery (unlawful touching) and for negligence (the failure to meet approved professional standards of care). The critical issue in the former is whether or not the patient, or in the case of children the person legally responsible for that child, has given informed consent to a procedure. Here we run into any manner of problems when adults are concerned and even more when we consider children.

Four general principles of ethics in medicine

A central principle is that of *autonomy*, defined in the *Oxford dictionary* as the right of self-government. One can elaborate that to see it as people's right to decide what they want and how they go about getting it. Although it is of enormous importance, the notion of autonomy cannot be allowed to be the only deciding factor in ethical matters. There must be added the proviso that society expects responsible behaviour from its members and in nine cases out of ten there will be other people involved in anyone's actions.

Adults may, along the way, think of others, their loved ones, their colleagues, their friends; they may even think of the doctor ('Oh, I wouldn't want to worry her with that'). However, in the final analysis it is the individual who is expected to decide whether or not to have medical treatment and what type of treatment to try to obtain, within financial constraints. Incidentally, we do not automatically give up our autonomy when we put ourselves in others' hands, whether those hands belong to a nurse, a doctor, an airline pilot, or a bus driver, providing we have voluntarily put ourselves in that position.

Within the concept of autonomy is the idea of respect for the person, the assumption that people will always wish to exercise their rights unless they say to the contrary. Respect for the person in hospital is most clearly seen when trouble is taken to ensure that a patient fully understands what he or she is consenting to. Harder to manage in many ways is the drawing of a line on the other side, of withholding information. Respect for others' rights to not always make decisions is sometimes called for, especially in paediatrics, and can be one of the hardest tests staff have to face. It may seem obvious that part of the process of informed consent is that truth is paramount. Should we always share everything and should we share it with everybody? It is not unknown for information to be given to the healthy husband or wife but not to their sick partner. This is a particular problem with children.

A second principle is that of doing good and avoiding harm, usually expressed as *beneficence and non-maleficence*. The oath and declarations at the beginning of this chapter all follow the general line that people practise medicine in order to do good, which can lead to doctors assuming that they have not only the right but the duty to make final decisions about treatment since they know best. We come now to another key phrase, 'best interests'. Medical staff may know all that anyone can about the effects of a certain drug or operation on a person, but they will never know all about that person in other ways. Even harder, they will never or only very rarely be able to perceive the world thorough their patients' eyes.

The third principle is that of *professional integrity* when we have to ask ourselves what the impact will be of what is done on the practice and profession of medicine. As Campbell *et al.* (1992) have pointed out, health care is not just an instant transaction but a growing body of expertise and shared skills, dependent on respectful relations between health workers.

Finally comes *justice*, by which is meant the fair allocation of resources. Are we discriminating between individuals on the basis of their medical need or on grounds of class, race, or wealth? At one level we can all argue that the latter criteria are to be condemned but resources are finite and some form of rationing or resource allocation is inevitable. This shades into a socio-political discussion which, while fascinating, is beyond the scope of this book. Anyone wishing to pursue the matter should consult Kennedy and Grubb (1994).

To live or to die

This is a stark heading but it has been chosen deliberately for there are times when people working in hospitals have to join in making stark choices. I say 'join in' since it is hoped that such decisions will be made by a number of people rather than one.

Those who feel that there may be times when children should be allowed to die generally invoke one or more of the moral principles outlined above to support their views. They look, for example, at a child who has no conscious appreciation of life and who is never likely to develop it. If such children are never likely to be able to be aware of the care and love of others then the principle of justice may come in, since resources spent on child A could be better used for child B, a notion known in economic theory as 'opportunity cost'. As Campbell *et al.* (1992) have put it, 'Our normal medical concern to treat for recovery can be appropriately suppressed.' They include in this group children with microcephaly, anencephaly, and certain other major central nervous system deformities.

A second group are those who have some capacity for human relationships but who have such severe handicaps that intervention to maintain life seems to do little more than prolong suffering. The decision in such cases is often to offer no more than basic comfort and custodial care.

A third group, related to the second but not quite identical, are those children whose treatment could so reduce their quality of life that on balance it is thought better that they should not live. Here I am thinking of an 8 year old with cancer who had endured treatment which had been nasty, brutish, and long. She was told that all that medicine had to offer was a drug which might extend her life by a few months but which would probably have unpleasant side-effects. 'It's my life', she said, 'I would rather be dead.' There is some support from a study published in the USA (Nitschke *et al.* 1982) for the conclusion that other young patients agree with this view.

Taking these arguments to their logical conclusion would lead to doctors sometimes not simply withholding treatment but actually killing children, as one would an animal in pain.

There are counter-arguments to these views. Singer (1983) points out that children are members of the species *Homo sapiens* and that this leads us to regard their needs as different from those we would ascribe to a dog or cat. What is more, many people depend on feelings rather than thoughts to provide the bedrock of the moral code on which ethics are built. Although we can talk about the rights and wrongs of any action, a tendency to empathize with other humans is built into our nature and some staff and parents have been trained or brought up to the idea, to think that all lives are sacred, that our concern for humans is a fundamental part of our nature as ethical beings, and that every possible effort should be made to keep everyone alive as long as possible. It is this belief, they say, which leads us to care for our young, come what may.

Others conclude that moral statements in this context are no more than an expression of emotion.

We are left with two extremes: keep everyone alive at all costs and thus, possibly, prolong the suffering of the patient and of the family or eliminate handicap and end suffering in a way that ignores some fundamental human impulses. If there were an easy answer there would be no need to discuss the matter.

Consent to treatment and to research

In adult medicine

The first point about consent is that it should be informed; information must be given to the patient (or parent) in such detail and in such a way that the person is in full possession of all the relevant facts.

This not inconsiderable task having been achieved, consent to treatment includes two components: first, agreement with a proposed aim related to improved health and, second, to the means of getting there, the treatment.

Sometimes it is easy. You are in a road accident, you break a leg, you are taken to hospital, given an X-ray, and put into plaster. Of course you give consent to all that, why on earth would you not?

Sometimes it is much harder. You are in hospital with what you know is a life-threatening illness and you are aware of a treatment that may or may not cure your condition, that may or may not have the most terrible side-effects.

Consent to research may also be easy, since it may involve no more than filling in a questionnaire on how one feels but in the context of hospital medicine research often involves patients taking part in a randomized controlled trial of different treatments.

In both treatment and research dilemmas one has to weigh the possible good with the possible harm, benefits against risks. The greater the benefits and the more serious the risks, the more we need to look to some under underlying principles of rights, duties, morals, and the law.

Consent in paediatrics

Most writing on the subject has wrestled with the question of when children can be expected to be competent. There is a tension between the need to respect children's liberties and adults' perception of the need for protection. Ethicists have frequently taken the somewhat arbitrary cut-off age of 16 years as one at which individuals can give consent but legislation in several parts of the world does not always concur. The Medical Research Council, in their report for the year 1962–1963, saw 12 years as a cut-off point above which competence to consent to research can be assumed to be based on comprehension.

English common law is vague about the age of consent to medical treatment, with a range from 16 years upwards for girls and 14 years upwards for boys. In Scotland the ages are 12 and 14 years. The Children Act, discussed below, causes further confusion. The critical feature of debates in this arena is the ability of children to understand what is at issue.

In the United States there is variation from state to state, with the notion of the mature minor coming into play in some. In Alabama the cut-off age is fixed at 14 years while in Mississippi the criterion is not age but competency to understand.

Nicholson (1986) saw two significant turning points: one was at the age of around 7 years when children's level of understanding makes it possible to communicate with them about health issues. The other comes at approximately 14 years when children's competence has developed to a level which enables them to make decisions about their health.

A challenging article recently appeared (Koren *et al.* 1993) in which the authors described out of class lessons in babysitting which included dealing with life-threatening emergencies. It was pointed out that there is a considerable discrepancy between the acknowledged responsibility of the 9–14 year olds when they are babysitting and the rights they enjoy to give consent to research.

The distinction between consent and assent is relevant here; the former implies full understanding, the latter implies no more than agreement. Nicholson's (1988) reasoning leads to the recommendation that assent be sought from children of 7 years and upwards and consent from the age of 14 years.

Bedevilling all this is the fact that one cannot really rely on age as a criterion since one child is so different from another. Nor can one use measured intelligence: the cognitive potential of a 9 year old may be similar to that of a child 5 years older but the second will have had so much more experience and may be more emotionally mature than the older one. Kennedy and Grubb (1994) argue against any notion of group membership as a determinant in decisions about understanding, putting forward the view that the concern of both ethics and the law is with the individual. They point out also that one should not confuse the general capacity to understand with actually understanding in a particular situation. For a continuation of the debate see the discussion of the Children Act, below.

Consent to paediatric research

The fundamental dilemma here is that unless research projects can be shown to be of direct benefit to an individual child, the guiding light of the child's best interest leads to a question about the validity of asking any child to take part without his or her fully informed consent. An extreme view is that all research on young children should be banned. An alternative approach is to broaden the notion of benefit to include general gain, as it were for all humanity.

The need to obtain young people's consent to research is thrown into sharp focus when the topic of the study is such that only young people can contribute as participants, an example being the use of antibiotics to treat sexually transmitted diseases in teenagers. The dilemma arises when it is evident that to ask parents for their consent would invade their children's privacy.

The American Academy of Pediatrics asserts that waiving parental consent is acceptable if the risks are minimal, if the question being asked by the study can be answered only if young people take part, and if the treatment leading from it will be available to young people with their consent only.

Campbell *et al.* (1992) have argued that we can countenance the involvement of children in research providing some stringent conditions are observed.

1. It can never be justified to volunteer another person to undergo any significant risk for what can be only an indirect benefit.

2. Parental consent does not, *ipso facto*, legitimize a research project.

3. Every effort should be made to ensure that the child is a participant rather than just a subject.

4. No research which could equally well be done on adults should be carried out on children.

Consent to treatment

This is a harder nettle to grasp partly because there is likely, by definition, to be some direct benefit to the children in question, unlike the case of research where benefit is more diffuse. If the notion of the invasion of privacy mentioned above leads to a reluctance to approach parents and, thus, the possibility that treatment is not given, an attempt at gaining consent from children themselves must be made.

Consent to treatment by proxy

There has recently been an explosion of interest in this topic, sparked off in part by the Children Act 1989, which is discussed later in this chapter. In some American states and in Australia the process is extended to adults who are unable to make decisions as well.

Strictly speaking, English law prevents parents from giving proxy consent to research which is of no direct benefit to the child but such research which affords 'no greater than minimal risk' has not, to date, been challenged in court.

One of the leading authors in the study of consent to treatment by proxy, Alderson (1990), has argued in her book that consent should be seen first of all as a two-way process: doctors give information and then the family not only seek clarification but also give information back, within the context of the repercussions on other family members. After all, consenting to a major procedure for one child can lead to massive effects on other members of the family: Mary has the operation but James has to stay with granny and Peter with his friend and Peter is taking exams in a month's time so is that the right place for him to be? What is more, parents have sometimes to think way ahead, to what their child might say in 10 years' time if a certain procedure is or is not carried out, a frequently occurring problem in plastic surgery. Informed consent which assumes that the participants can have knowledge of the future is for many people and in many situations an impossibility.

Implicit in this approach is the idea that one has to get away from the one-off talk leading to a decision; some aspects of complex treatment may take several hours spread over several days before everyone is satisfied that the groundwork has been covered.

Implicit also in the notion of a family–doctor process is the idea of involving a team: as far as possible the child should take part as well.

Alderson (1990) sees three threads running through proxy consent. The first is emotions. 'Deciding about risky surgery involves deeply feeling fear, hope, anguish and trust. Strong ambivalent feeling also continues well after a decision is made.' As she points out, it would be odd if parents of a sick child were not anxious. Gouldner (1977) has discussed two forms of knowledge: that which is understood solely at an intellectual level and that which is awareness, working at mental, physical, and emotional levels. The law and perhaps many doctors tend to work within one type while parents are likely to be at least for part of the time at the second type.

Secondly, there is the issue of the imbalance in power between staff and parents. Hospitals are often large and usually complex organizations and it is easy to underestimate how intimidating they can be to those who do not work in one. If the system gives the message that it is all-powerful, that the individual parent or patient is of little significance, there will be a further message that when major matters of consent are under consideration the system will override all else.

The third thread is related to the second: practical details in the design and running of a ward may facilitate or impede parental inter-action with ward staff. A ward or unit in which parents feel at home and welcome is likely to provide a setting more conducive to the process of decision making than one where parents constantly feel that they are perceived as interlopers.

The components of proxy consent

Informed proxy consent depends on parents both being given and understanding adequate medical information.

Alderson (1990) has postulated seven components.

1. Voluntary proxy consent depends on parents being able to make decisions freely.

2. Adequate or good-enough consent describes a realistic approach towards helping parents to make as informed and free a choice as possible.

3. Proxy consent assesses harm and benefit, not as abstractions but as physical and mental experiences.

4. Proxy consent may involve drawing a line.

5. Proxy consent is both a formal agreement and a process.

6. Proxy consent includes understanding, choosing, knowing that it is possible to refuse, and signifying the decision.

7. Proxy consent has to be seen in the context of how each hospital encourages or restricts family-centred care.

The consent form

Some take the signing of the consent form seriously, while some regard it as a formality to get through. I was struck, some years ago, to discover that the majority of parents attending a hospital parents' group claimed to have no recollection of ever having signed such a form. A recent study (Byrne *et al.* 1988) published in the *British Medical Journal* found that 40 per cent of the patients who had signed a consent form had very little idea about what they had signed for. If there is no evidence that consent was informed the document is legally of no value. And yet it stands for so much and if it is not signed the procedure cannot take place. As with so much, it is not just the piece of paper that is of value, it is the discussion that goes on around it.

The right to refuse treatment

An immensely tricky question arises not only with consent to treatment but to the right to refuse. American law in some states gives parents the right to consent to medical care for their dependent children but not the co-equal right to refuse care deemed medically necessary. (See also the discussion below on minors' right to refuse.)

Jehovah's Witnesses

Jehovah's Witnesses are Christians who see the Bible as a source of guidance throughout life. They quote Leviticus 17: 13, 14 as forbidding the partaking of the blood of any flesh: 'Anyone who partakes of it shall be cut off.' This applies even in a medical emergency involving the possible loss of life and applies to all blood, even one's own. Red cells, white cells, platelets, and blood plasma are all forbidden.

There are alternatives to blood products, saline solutions for example, but it happens from time to time that the responsible clinician will be of the opinion that only the giving of blood will save a patient's life. A number of hospitals have drawn up guidelines on this topic; those quoted below are from the document drawn up in Great Ormond Street.

1. Decisions should ideally be taken only after ample discussion with everyone concerned.

2. A distinction should be made between:

    a. An acute emergency when there may be no time to discuss with anyone.

    b. An emergency when there is time to discuss but not to refer elsewhere.

    c. Elective procedures when there is time to discuss and possibly to refer elsewhere if necessary.

3. It has been found helpful to elicit Witnesses' concepts of God's view of punishment; if they can be reassured that they have done their utmost to avoid the partaking of blood then they, and the hospital staff, are more likely to be comfortable when the procedure occurs.

If parents or patients are adamant about not giving consent, a record of their refusal should be entered into the child's notes, signed by them and the doctor and colleagues.

A graphic example of this came with a 12 year old Jehovah's Witness who was as unhappy as his parents at the thought of receiving a transfusion. The nursing staff were also reluctant in the extreme to take part in this aspect of his treatment. The solution came after hours of discussion from which it was learnt that he believed that providing people strive to their utmost to do right they are not punished for any transgression of the holy law. He then made a signed declaration, put into the medical notes, to the effect that he did not wish to receive any blood products. It was explained to him that he *would* have them if it was thought necessary but that in this way everyone would know that the treatment was against his will. When the time came for the transfusion he was quite calm and he and his parents remained on good terms with the staff.

4. When parents refuse to go ahead an alternative clinician should, if possible, be recommended to the family.

5. It is not generally necessary to apply for the removal of a child from parental custody. In Britain, section 8 of the Children Act 1989 is seen as a basis for such removal but this has been challenged by recent cases. If it is thought that legal steps may be needed, the hospital's social services department should be consulted. (If the problem is as extreme as that the hospital social services should have been involved from a much earlier stage.)

6. It is worth noting a Witness's greatest fear is that they will be given blood while unconscious.

7. A valuable step, when there is doubt, is to consult the Witness's liaison service which is available 24 hours a day.

It is sometimes assumed that a Jehovah's Witness's family will reject a child who has been given blood as unclean. In fact, there is no recorded case of this having happened.

Confidentiality

There are clear guidelines on confidentiality; quoted below are points based on those laid down by the General Medical Council.

The doctor is responsible to the patient or person with whom there is a professional relationship for the security and confidentiality of information given.

A doctor must preserve secrecy with five exceptions.

1. When the patient gives consent.

2. When it is undesirable on medical grounds to seek a patient's consent but it is in the patient's own interest that confidentiality is broken.

3. When the doctor's overriding duty to society is seen as more important.

4. For the purpose of medical research, when approved by the relevant ethical committee.

5. When the information is required by due legal process.

The Children Act 1989

The Children Act 1989 is addressed mainly to the court and local authority social services departments but contains a good deal which has, potentially at least, immense implications for the care of children in hospital. It replaced almost all the previous legislation about children with a single, coherent framework aiming to simplify the legal position of children. For the first time private law (relating to the way individuals behave towards each other) and public law (which deals with those areas where society intervenes in the lives of individuals) are brought together.

The key concept is that the child's welfare is the paramount consideration of the court. However, 'welfare', 'best interest', and all such phrases are invariably defined by adults.

Secondly, there is a new concept of parental responsibility, to replace parental rights. This responsibility is lost only when a child is adopted. Parents now have new rights to a say in plans being made for their child's future. Unmarried fathers may obtain parental responsibility by agreement or by a court order.

Definitions of children in need are also spelled out as are those related to the notion of significant harm, which can include the impairment of physical, intellectual, emotional, social, or behavioural development.

There is a new framework for the care and protection of children, rationalizing the grounds on which a court can make care and supervision orders.

The first item on a check-list of factors which the court must consider before reaching a decision about a child is the duty to ascertain the wishes and feelings of the child, with consideration for the age and understanding of the child but no stated age limitations. The child's age, gender, health, personality, race, culture, life, and experiences are all relevant to any consideration of needs and have to be taken into account when planning or providing help.

Of particular relevance to children in hospital are the new duties that the local authority has, to ensure that the welfare of children who are being looked after away from home, including those in hospital, is safeguarded. Health authorities intending to look after a child for more than 3 months have to inform the local social services department and must also give notice when the child leaves.

Within the context of consent to treatment one can see the possible ramifications of the philosophy underlying this extremely important legislation. If it is deemed that a child is capable of understanding, then that child could, possibly even should, be expected to be a party not only to assent to treatment but also to consent.

In 1970 Lord Denning spoke of 'parents' dwindling right which the court will hesitate to enforce against the wishes of the child' (Lord Justice Denning, Hewer vs Bryant 1970 1 QB 357, 369). More recently the Gillick case is invariably quoted whenever a minor's consent is discussed. This case involved the right of a doctor to prescribe contraceptives to a young person under the age of 16 years without parental consent (Gillick vs West Norfolk & Wisbech AHA (1985) 3 All ER 402 (1985) 2BMLR 11 (HL)). The ruling indicated that parental rights to determine whether or not their child below the age of 16 years will have medical treatment terminates, 'if and when the child achieves a sufficient understanding and intelligence to enable him or her to understand fully what is proposed'.

The Law Lords' ruling on Gillick lead to the coining of the phrase, 'Gillick competent child', defined as 'one who achieves a sufficient understanding and intelligence to enable him or her to make a wise choice in his or her own interests'. See Alderson (1993) and Kennedy and Grubb (1994) for a fuller discussion of this case and of children's consent in general.

Children's rights to refuse treatment

A quite different matter is the child's right to refuse treatment. The Children Act 1989 states that when a court orders an assessment, 'if the child is of sufficient understanding to make an informed decision he may refuse to submit to a medical or psychiatric examination or other assessment' (Part V, section 43(8)).

It should be noted here that the act is primarily about children in need of local authority services rather than about those in hospital. Nevertheless, I have known one case in which a 10 year old refused to have an operation. His parents wanted him to have it but there was no overwhelming medical reason for operating and the surgeon upheld the child's right to say no.

In practice the law says differently. In two recent cases the Court of Appeal has made it clear that the right to withhold consent to treatment by children under the age of 18 years is not comparable to their right to give consent (Korgaonkar and Tribe 1993). It is to be noted that both cases concerned children in need of or arguably in need of psychiatric care and it is possible that the issue of their competence to withhold consent affected the court's decision.

The judgement by Lord Donaldson on one of these cases concluded that 'Lord Scarman cannot have been intending to say that the parental right to consent terminates with the achievement by the child of Gillick competence.' Lawyers and others have argued furiously about Lord Donaldson's pronouncement (Alderson 1993) but the 1992 judgement in the High Court of the case of W, a minor, has led the Lord Chancellor's Department (personal communication) to the conclusion that 'no minor of whatever age has power by refusing consent to treatment to override the consent given by anyone else who has parental responsibility in respect of him (or her)'.

In other words, children's views are to be upheld as long as they say yes. No doubt the debate will continue.

The protection of children

It was noted above that there is often a tension between the need to uphold the rights of children and the need to protect them and three new child protection orders have been created by the Children Act 1989, all of which may at times be relevant for children in hospital:

(1) a child assessment order;

(2) an emergency protection order;

(3) a recovery order.

Health professionals are most likely to be involved with the first of these which is covered in section 43 of the act. It is made where significant harm is suspected but the child is not thought to be at immediate risk. It can also be made when the social services department or some authorized person considers that an assessment is required; the parent(s) or person responsible for the child has refused to cooperate and the court has found that all reasonable steps to persuade those caring for the child have been taken. Those responsible for the child should be warned that a child assessment order may be applied for if they continue to fail to cooperate. (An authorized person in this context is one authorized by the Secretary of State to bring proceedings under section 31 of the act. This covers the NSPCC and its officers.)

As its name implies, its purpose is to allow the social services department or other authorized person, to find out more about the child's health or development or the way that he/she has been treated in order to decide what further action may be required.

An order may be made when the court is satisfied on one of the following.

1. That there is reasonable cause to suspect that the child is suffering or is likely to suffer significant harm.

2. That there are good grounds for carrying out an assessment of the child's health or development in order to determine whether he/she is suffering or is likely to suffer significant harm.

The order is made for a maximum of 7 days and leads to a compulsion on the part of the parent or person responsible for the child to produce him/her to the person named in the order so that the assessment may be made. Refusal to comply is usually seen as sufficient grounds for an emergency protection order (see below).

A number of points arise in connection with the practice of this procedure. It should be used sparingly, only when there is serious concern, and not in cases of emergency. It is usually most appropriate when the harm to the child is thought to be long-term and cumulative rather than sudden and severe. It should also be noted that the court will direct on the limits and scope of the assessment, the criteria, and the methods and developmental tools to be used.

From this it will be seen that people working in hospitals have a duty to alert the social services department if there is anxiety about, for example, a child who is failing to thrive, the possibility of abuse or neglect, or when an assessment is needed to establish basic facts about a child's condition and staff are hindered in carrying out this assessment.

The normal procedure is for the social worker concerned to call a case conference under local child protection procedures. The person voicing anxiety will have to contribute to this conference, as will anyone else who has significant dealings with the child or family.

Persistent refusal to allow a child to be seen rings warning bells and is usually sufficient to warrant applying for an emergency protection order under the 'frustrated access' condition.

Careful plans should be made to allow the full assessment to be made within the 7 days of the order.

A child judged to be capable of understanding the consequences may consent or refuse assessment. A decision will then have to be made about the next step following investigation by a guardian *ad litem*. (A guardian *ad litem* is someone appointed by the court to investigate a child's circumstances and present a non-partisan view of the child's welfare to the court.)

An emergency protection order

This is what its name implies: it is a short-term order (maximum 8 days which may be extended once only by a further 7 days) which enables a child to be made safe when there is reasonable cause to believe that the child is likely to suffer significant harm. It replaces the old Place of Safety Order.

Although in theory anyone can apply for an emergency order, in practice it will be the social services department or an authorized person. A crucial factor is that applications can be made without notice of the hearing having been given to anyone else.

The act is still recent enough for there to be a lack of case law supporting its interpretation.

Rights of access to medical records

I had explained to my 13 year old patient that I needed to make notes of our conversation because I might otherwise forget the details of what had been said. She was happy with this but at the end of the session asked, politely, if she might see what I had written. As I handed the page over to her she added that she knew that since November 1991 she had a right to seem them anyway. She was, of course, correct.

The 1984 Data Protection Act gave individuals the right of access to all computerized health and other records; the 1990 Access to Health Records Act gave patients right of access to their manually held health records made on or after 1 November 1991.

What that means in practice is that all National Health Service and private patients in England, Wales, and Scotland may apply to examine and obtain copies of the whole or extracts from any records relating to their mental or physical health and they will be able to ask that corrections be made to those records. If the professional who was responsible for them disagrees about the correction he or she has a duty to add a note to the effect that the patient considers the entry to be incorrect. The act applies only to those records made by a professional in connection with that individual who is making the application. Health professional in this context includes, among others, registered nurses, midwives, chiropodists, dieticians, and speech therapists.

Anyone wishing to gain access to notes must apply in writing to the holder of the record, likely to be a general practitioner or the hospital concerned. The health authority or trust or whoever is the holder, must then seek the advice of the professional involved before making a decision on whether to give access or not. There is generally not likely to be any reason for withholding information but the case might arise that to give full access would reveal data about a third party which the professional feels should remain confidential to that person. It is also possible to withhold information if it is thought that giving it would cause serious harm to the person's physical or mental health or that of another person. If it is agreed to give access this must be granted within 40 days of receipt of the written application.

Children under 16 years may apply but this request will be granted only if the holder of the record is satisfied that the young person understands the import of the application. Parents or guardians may apply as well but once again this will be acceded to only if the holding authority is satisfied either that the child has given consent or is unable to understand the nature of the application and that to grant it would be in that child's best interests. (This applies also to adults who are unable to manage their own affairs.) If the child has expressly requested that whatever is said during an interview remain confidential or if it is clear that this was the child's understanding, the records should not be made available to others without that child's permission. This is of great importance in areas of child abuse or family planning.

When the application is made on behalf of a child or adult, the holders have the right to release only those parts of the notes that apply to the person concerned.

This is not all: once the records have been seen the patient may ask for a copy of them and for an explanation of any part that is not understood. This is seen to refer not so much to medical terminology but more to illegible handwriting.

A declaration on the rights of children in institutions

In 1992 four people came together at the request of the International Association of Child and Adolescent Psychiatry and Allied Professions to contribute to a debate on the rights of children in institutions. These four drew up the declaration given below; it reflects their personal views and should not be quoted as representing their employers or the Association.

The rights of children in institutions

1. Preamble

The Convention on the Rights of the Child, adopted by the General Assembly of the United Nations on 20 November 1989, is a backdrop to the statements that follow.

It is acknowledged that:

The primary consideration is the best interests of the child at all times.

All children should enjoy the highest possible standards of safety, health care and education.

All children have a common right of access to a developmental pathway leading to the maximum possible productive adult citizenship consistent with their individual capacities.

Children are of equal worth, whatever their race, ability, gender, sexual orientation, social class or religion.

Society should recognise the needs and characteristics of children at different stages and respond appropriately to them.

Children deserve respect.

Separation of children from their family should occur only to ensure the children's well being.

If children are separated from their family and are living in institutions both should know where the other is. They should also have access to each other and be able to communicate with each other.

Children are the responsibility of society as a whole. Residential care must be perceived as a valued, important activity.

2. *Definition of a child*

A child is anyone below the age of 18 years unless the local law of majority is different.

3. *Definition of an institution*

Any out of home establishment in which children live.
Included are:
Boarding schools (Independent, State and those for children with
    special educational needs)
Local Authority children's homes
Voluntary and private children's homes
Intermediate Treatment Units
Youth Treatment Centres
Establishments for Youth Custody
Hospitals, including Adolescent Units
The Armed Services.

The range of provision noted above will mean that some of the statements made below are more pertinent in one setting than another. Nevertheless, as far as possible general principles have been addressed.

4. Limitations on the role of the institution

It is acknowledged that, as far as possible and feasible, institutions should act as partners with parents in their care of children. Boundaries of care will vary according to the nature of the institution and the characteristics of the child.

5. Accommodation

Children should live in a setting that is comfortable, safe and geared to their needs.

6. Protection from abuse

Children should be protected from physical and emotional harm, economic exploitation, deprivation or disadvantage, whether such harm is at the hands of an individual or a system.

7. Protection from distress

Steps should be taken to mitigate children's physical or emotional distress. Their privacy should be respected.

8. Limitations on safeguards

It is easy to consider rights of children in terms of their protection. Less often discussed, but not unimportant, is the right of all children to take reasonable risks in order that they should grow.

9. The views of children

The value of children's own views and perceptions should be recognised and fully taken into account in any decisions relating to their care, management or treatment, bearing in mind their age and abilities.

10. Access to information

Children should be able to seek and receive information from the mass media and from communication with individuals by letter, telephone or any other means, consistent with their health and safety and the rights of others.

11. Freedom of expression

It is acknowledged that in many cases the cultural background of the children will differ from that of those who care for them. Nevertheless, carers should understand the culture of the children for whom they are responsible, reflecting it generally, enabling children to express an opinion, to speak a language, partake in cultural activities and practise religious beliefs which are consistent with the children's health and safety and the rights of others.

12. Sexual feelings

Children deserve respect for their sexual feelings.

13. Knowledge of the rules and expectations of the institution

Children should be made aware of the rules and expectations of the institution in which they find themselves and should have access to someone in authority who can explain the rules to them.

14. Personal communication within and without the institution

a) There should be a named person within each institution, whose role it is to take a personal interest in individual children.
b) There should also be a named person outside each institution to whom individual children have ready access.
c) There should be a clear channel of communication so that complaints may be heard and allegations about deficiencies in care investigated. The named person mentioned in section b) above should be involved in this procedure.

15. Staff

a) Those responsible for caring for children should have adequate knowledge and skills to fulfil their role, should receive sufficient supervision to ensure that their work is carried on to the highest possible level and should have access to external advice on matters both general and specific.
b) All staff should have high expectations of children in their care.

16. Children's development

Children have the right to rest, play, recreation, intellectual stimulation, physical activity and the fostering of talents.

17. Sanctions

Children should not receive corporal punishment. Sanctions should not involve depriving them of basic rights, for example to food, health care, education or access to their parents.

18. Reviews of placements

There should be periodic reviews of all children's placements bearing in mind their needs for education, health care and general development.

19. Continuity and predictability

Children need continuity in care and a predictable environment. At a macro level this implies as few changes as possible in their overall management; at a micro level it signals a need for daily and longer term stability in the people looking after them.

Contributors to this statement

David Berridge	Research & Development Director, National Children's Bureau, London
Lesley Hollinshead	Child Care Training Officer, London Borough of Greenwich Social Services Department
Jack Ind	Formerly Headmaster of Dover College, Kent
Richard Lansdown	Consultant Psychologist, The Hospital for Sick Children, London

The making of video tapes in hospital

The widespread use of video for clinical and teaching purposes is not without its legal and ethical hazards. Great Ormond Street Hospital has produced guidelines which are given in full in Appendix 3.

References

Alderson, P. (1990). *Choosing for children*. Oxford University Press, Oxford.
Alderson, P. (1993). *Children's consent to surgery*. Open University Press, Buckingham.

Byrne, D., Napier A., and Cushieri, A. (1988). How informed is signed consent? *British Medical Journal*, **296**, 839–41.

Campbell, A., Gillett, G., and Jones, G. (1992). *Practical medical ethics*. Oxford University Press, Auckland.

Faulder, C. (1985). *Whose body is it?* Virago Press, London.

Gouldner, A. (1977). *The coming crisis in Western sociology*. Heinemann, London.

Kennedy, I. and Grubb, A. (1994). Medical law: text with materials. (Second edition). Butterworths, London.

Koren, G., Carmeli, D.B., Carmeli, Y.S., and Haslam, R. (1993). Maturity of children to consent to medical research: the baby sitter test. *Journal of Medical Ethics*, **19**, 142–7.

Nicholson, R. (1986). *Medical research with children: ethics, law and practice*. Oxford University Press, Oxford.

Nitschke, R., Humphrey, G.B., Ssexauer, C.L., Catron, B., Wunder, S., and Jay, S. (1982). Therapeutic choices made by patients with end-stage cancer. *Journal of Pediatrics*, **101**, 471–6.

Singer, P. (1983). Sanctity of life of quality of life? *Pediatrics*, **72**, 274–8.

21

The hospital of tomorrow

There is an understandable tendency to predict the future within the framework of the present; more of what we have now will lead to such and such a development. I have no crystal ball and so I will follow this tradition and look at what might happen in the light of recent developments. A transformation in hospitals could come from four sources. The first is a shift in practice, the second is the development of technology, the third the interest among architects in linking buildings with health care in a more direct way than hitherto, and the fourth is the need to save money.

Changes in practice

Paediatric community nursing services

Care at home has been the first choice ever since the 1959 Platt Report stated that children should be admitted to hospital only if the care they require cannot be as well provided at home. The 1991 Department of Health Report *The welfare of children and young people in hospital* repeated the message.

The first paediatric community nursing scheme in Britain was set up in 1948 in Rotherham and although the growth was slow at first, by 1992 there were 52 schemes with 30 specialist teams caring for children with specific diseases. The average length of stay of children in hospital is now only 2 days and, as is discussed in Chapter 3, there has been a rise in day case admissions.

Care by parent

This is a logical extension of what has happened over parents visiting in hospital: first they were excluded, then they were allowed in for a few hours a week, after which they were welcomed, as visitors, at any time. The Care by Parent scheme welcomes them as carers, not just as visitors. The idea that this practice is new could be regarded with some cynicism by anyone who has been to a hospital in a developing country where parents frequently care for their children. The idea that it is that new in more developed countries is scotched when one realizes that there was a feasibility study in the United States in 1960 on the setting up of a domiciliary centre for children who did not need conventional care but needed to attend hospital for treatment, procedures, or evaluation (Green and Segar 1961).

We should distinguish between two groups of children. The first are those referred to in the paragraph above; those who could just as well stay in a nearby hotel, being looked after by their parents, attending hospital only for their medical care. It is possible to imagine a hospital of the future that will have a hotel built alongside, not only for parents and patients but for siblings and other family members as well. The success of accommodation already provided on a small scale for families, the Ronald MacDonald houses in America and the Sick Children's Trust accommodation in London, shows that this is likely to be welcomed by families who come from some distance.

The second group are those children who must, for medical reasons, remain on a ward but whose medical needs can be met, to a large extent, by their parents. These parents have, of course, to be taught by nursing staff and there has to be a nurse readily available in times of crisis but it has been shown that parents can undertake medical procedures that might have been thought the sole prerogative of the nurse. Staff in Cardiff came up with four levels of care that parents might perform, ranging from general child care that was common to all parents to advanced nursing which included feeding by nasogastric tube and physiotherapy (Bromley 1992). I have known many parents who have become competent in dealing with a Hickman catheter.

There are some difficulties of course. Some parents may not feel that they are competent enough to undertake complex procedures. If there are some children on a ward who are cared for more or less completely by their parents and others are not, this may make the parents of the second group feel inferior. For this reason it has been suggested that units be all or nothing; care by nurse or care by parent. Some parents are uneasy because they feel that they are doing nurses out of a job, while some nurses are wary of entrusting even oral medication to parents (Webb *et al.* 1985).

Another difficulty is deciding not only which parents are capable but which patients are suitable for care by parent. Goodband and Jennings (1992) put forward 20 situations, including parents who need to develop skills in certain procedures before children can be discharged; the authors give gastrostomies and tracheostomies as examples, newly diagnosed chronic illnesses such as diabetes and cystic fibrosis, when blind or deaf children are in hospital, and the child with cardiac problems who needs continued observation, medication, and monitoring of weight gain.

The economic argument for this approach is appealing: in Canada, Evans and Robinson (1983) found that a parent care unit's costs were 33 per cent lower than those of a general paediatric ward, 13.5 per cent lower for tonsil and adenoid surgery and 29 per cent lower for other surgery. What is more, the average length of stay was 25 per cent shorter.

The development of technology

There are two key features here. The advances in fibre optic transmission, leading to an ability to transmit clear pictures, combined with the miniaturization of equipment, has given rise to the rapidly developing facility to transmit information from one place to another with an accuracy and detail that has never before been known. The second feature is that this technology could soon be available to all hospitals and to general practitioners in local health centres, so it is or soon will be possible for a child to go to a local centre for an X-ray and for the image to be transmitted to a specialist in a teaching hospital in a matter of seconds. Satellite image acquisition, due soon, means that there is likely to be a world-wide, integrated voice–data–video communication system. There will still be a need to admit some children for some investigations but a large proportion of what can now be done in only a few places, mainly because they are where the expertise is found, will be carried out at long range.

Design and health

Although medical, social, and political changes are so rapid in many countries that there is much to be said for designing buildings with little more than a 10 year life, this is such an impractical idea that it is unlikely ever to be followed to the letter. However, there might be a degree of flexibility built into hospital design, to allow for changes, for example, with much larger out-patient areas should the present pattern of short admissions continue.

Scher (1992) began his paper on environmental design quality in health care by asserting that this topic has risen to the top of the agenda in Britain recently for three reasons.

The first is what he sees as an active dislike of the character and quality of the majority of new National Health Services hospital buildings as perceived by the patients, staff, and visitors. Too often, newly built environments are 'ugly, inhuman, mechanical, cold and cheerless'. Two qualifications have to be made here. One is that Scher (1992) was writing of hospitals in general; it would be unwise immediately to generalize to paediatric wards or units. The second is that he admits that this statement cannot be demonstrated for a significantly large number of people.

However, he goes on to make the point that up to now, design specifications have been related to functional fit and control of capital; there have been no specifications for warm and friendly designs. There are parallels in local authority housing designs, although it must be said that public outcry has seen the end at least of the tower block.

Second comes the interest of the Prince of Wales who, in a speech at the Royal Society of Medicine in 1990, linked good architectural design with healing.

Third is the specification of environmental quality in the new NHS contracts. The internal market structure allows contracts to embody conditions for environmental quality which have to be met. Whether purchasers will see expenditure on environmentally friendly design as worthwhile will remain to be seen.

Despite the endorsement by the Prince of Wales, there is very little research evidence to support the idea that the physical environment can influence the healing process. There is one study always quoted, that of Ulrich (1984), who produced data to show that a sample of 23 adult patients who had a room with a pleasant view recovered quicker than those whose room looked out onto a brick wall. The need for further work in this area, to encompass the well-being of staff as well as patients, is considerable.

Moss (1987) has differentiated between curing, healing, and caring. The first is the province of hospital staff, not of architects and designers. The second, however, is more broadly based since healing is something which takes place rather than being something which is administered. Caring 'is concerned to provide a tolerable level of physical and emotional comfort in difficult circumstances, so that healing may take place more easily'. Moss (1987) argued that we should not try to separate these three for all contribute to the restoration of health.

There have been some attempts to create friendly buildings. St Mary's on the Isle of Wight has its physical environment enhanced by well over 1000 works of art, from mosaics to engraved glass to tapestries to paintings. The Arts for Health Centre at Manchester is in the forefront of the thinking that led to much of St Mary's.

There can, of course, be attention to existing buildings as well. The anxious parent or staff member, lost in a maze of corridors, welcomes adequate indications of where departments and wards are, but how many hospitals are really well signposted? The introduction of the visual arts on paediatric wards has long given an example to adult hospitals, but it was not that long ago that a consultant in a London teaching hospital tore down children's paintings from a wall, exclaiming, 'This is a hospital, not a nursery school.'

Economic considerations

The need to save money runs through the British health service at the moment. In this Britain is not alone. It could be seen as a brake on some of the more imaginative schemes of architects and designers but in one way it could underpin a revolution in hospital provision. Keeping a child and parent(s) in a hospital is very expensive. As has been mentioned above, new technology may mean much more long-range consultation and a reduction in the need to have children sent to major centres for investigation but it is now realized that it is often not necesary for them to sleep in a hospital either, nor for their care be totally in the hands of qualified nurses.

References

Bromley, C. (1992). Developments in the Cardiff care-by-parent scheme. In *Caring for children in hospital*, (ed. J. Cleary). Scutari Press, London.

Evans, R.G. and Robinson, G.C. (1983). An economic study of cost savings on a care-by-parent ward. *Medical Care*, **21**, 768–82.

Goodband, S. and Jennings, K. (1992). Parent care: a US experience in Indianapolis. In *Caring for children in hospital*, (ed. J. Cleary). Scutari Press, London.

Green, M. and Segar, W.E. (1961). A new design for patient care and pediatric education in a children's hospital: an interim report. *Pediatrics*, **28**, 825–37.

Moss, L. (1987). *Art for health's sake*. Hospital Arts, Manchester. The Carnegie United Kingdom Trust.

Scher, P. (1992). *Environmental design quality in health care*. Arts for Health, Manchester Metropolitan University, Manchester.

Ulrich, R. (1984). View through a window may influence recovery from surgery. *Science*, **224**, 420–1.

Webb N., Hull, D., and Madeley, R. (1985). Care by parents in hospital. *British Medical Journal*, **291**, 176–7.

Appendix 1: Specialist children's dispensaries and hospitals founded in Britain during the 19th century

1816   London: Dr John Bunnell Davis's Universal Dispensary for Children
1820   London: Royal Western Infirmary Dispensary for Children
1821   Dublin: The National Children's Hospital
1829   Manchester: General Dispensary for Children
1840   London: Kensington Dispensary for Children
1851   Liverpool: Institution for the Diseases of Children
1852   London: The Great Ormond Street Hospital for Children (called for many years the Hospital for Sick Children)
1853   Norwich: Jenny Lind Children's Hospital
1855   Manchester: The General Hospital and Dispensary for Sick Children (developed from the dispensary opened in 1829)
1857   Liverpool: Children's Hospital
        Bristol: Children's Dispensary
        Leeds: Hospital for Women (and Children)
1860   Edinburgh: Royal Hospital for Children
1862   Birmingham: Children's Hospital
        Newcastle: Children's Hospital
1863   London: Belgrave Children's Hospital
1864   Sunderland: Children's Hospital
1866   London: Grosvenor Children's Hospital
        Victoria Hospital for Children, Chelsea
1867   London: Queen Elizabeth Hospital for Children (originally the North Eastern Hospital for Children)
        Gloucester: Children's Hospital
        London: Alexandra Hip Hospital, Queen Square
1868   London: East London Hospital for Children, Shadwell
        Brighton: Children's Hospital

1869   London: Evalina Children's Hospital
       Nottingham: Children's Hospital
       Birkenhead: Children's Hospital
1872   London: Sydenham Road Children's Hospital
       Hull: Children's Hospital
       Sevenoaks Children's Hospital
1873   Belfast: The Royal Hospital for Sick Children
1874   London: Cheyne Children's Hospital, Chelsea
       Cheltenham Children's Hospital
1876   Sheffield Children's Hospital
1883   London: Paddington Green Children's Hospital
       Bradford: Children's Hospital
       Glasgow: Royal Glasgow Hospital for Sick Children
1885   Bristol: Children's Hospital
1886   Newbury: Children's Hospital
1887   Gateshead: Children's Hospital
1888   Torquay: Rosehill Children's Hospital
1893   London: St Mary's Hospital for Children, Plaistow
1897   Aberdeen: Royal Hospital for Children
1899   Liverpool: Royal Liverpool Country Hospital for Children

Data from F.N.L. Poynter (ed) (1964) *The evolution of hospitals in Britain.* Pitman Medical Publishing, London.

Appendix 2: Ethical aspects of the use of videotaped recordings

The following notes are taken, with permission, from the policy guidelines issued by Great Ormond Street Hospital and the London Borough of Camden.

1. The primary purpose of all records is to enable professionals to manage the case as effectively as possible.

2. From November 1991 patients have the right to see their own case notes and the potential right to see video tapes made of interviews of themselves. Child patients cannot make an application unless the hospital be satisfied that the child is capable of understanding the nature of such an application.

   Access can be refused if, in the opinion of the holder of the record, it would disclose either
   a. Information likely to cause serious harm to the health of the patient or any other individual or
   b. Information relating to or provided by an individual other than the patient who could be identified from that information.

3. Where a request for the release of recordings for the purpose of legal proceedings is received the first step is for the hospital to show the recordings to the police or other authorities having a professional responsibility for the care of the child or for legal proceedings.

4. Release of the recordings from the custody of the hospital must only be by Court Order.

5. Disclosure to a person or body with parental responsibility should be determined by the hospital's view on whether this is desirable in the interests of the treatment of the child.

6. Disclosure for teaching or research purposes should only be with the written consent of the child patient concerned (if of sufficient understanding) and/or of the person or body with legal responsibility for the child.

7. Whenever possible there should be a full and open discussion about the possible implications of a video tape recording with the patient (if of sufficient understanding) and/or of the person or body when legal responsibility for the child. Written consent should be obtained and the consent form kept in the box containing the tape with a photocopy held elsewhere.

8. Copyright of all recordings is held by the hospital.

9. Written permission must be obtained from all members of staff involved in the case each time a tape is shown, e.g. for teaching purposes.

10. All tapes should be kept in a locked cupboard or filing cabinet in a locked room.

Appendix 3: Guidelines on child protection

The following notes have been compiled from a document entitled *Child protection policy, procedures and guidance*, issued by the Great Ormond Street Hospital for Children NHS Trust (1995).

1. In all cases the welfare, well-being and protection of the child has to be paramount.

2. It is vital that professionals make no lasting assumptions either that abuse must have taken place or that it never could.

3. The effective management of child abuse demands a multidisciplinary approach with consultation and exchange of information at every stage.

4. Any member of staff having concern about actual or possible abuse of any kind must inform the consultant or deputy and the senior nurse responsible for the ward/department. The social work department of the hospital *must* immediately be informed of any concern.

5. When suspicions of abuse are aroused by a specific presentation, the child's general physical health, emotional state, and behavioural state should be assessed.

6. The following four categories are used to register children's names on Local Authority Child Protection Registers: persistent or severe neglect; physical injury, actual or likely; sexual abuse, actual or likely; or sexual exploitation of a child or adolescent; and emotional abuse, actual or likely.

7. The following presentation of injuries or states which should alert concern include the following.

   (a) Inconsistencies between the account of injuries being incurred with their appearance and nature.
   (b) Timing of injuries being discrepant with the account given.
   (c) Indications of a series of injuries.

   (d) Unexplained injuries noted by others, for example in school.

   (e) An unusual degree of hostility or overfriendliness towards hospital staff.

   (f) An unusual lack of concern at the injuries.

8. Behavioural signs which may alert concern include the following.

   (a) Frozen watchfulness.

   (b) Playing/acting out in aggressive, highly active ways.

   (c) Unusual degrees of closeness or distance between parents and children.

9. If there are suspicions of Munchausen syndrome by proxy concerns should not be discussed with the parents in the first instance. The matter should be raised as in part 4 above.

10. The statutory duty for investigating any suspected child abuse lies with the social service department acting for the local authority and the Police Child Protection Team.

Index

boredom 40, 66
Boswell, James 4
bowel disorders 142
Bowlby, John 19–20
breast-feeding 17, 22
British Association for Counselling 163
British Medical Association 208, 211
Brook Hospital 68
Buchan, William 2, 6
building design 246–8
burn-out 203–4
burns 112

cancer 89, 139
  ethical issues 224
  inappropriate focus on stress-reduction 144
  stress among staff 216–18
Care by Parent scheme 244–6
catheters
  cardiac 112
  Hickman lines 78, 113, 243
Celsus, Cornelius 2
cerebral palsy 91
challenging 173–4
chaplains 196
charter for children in hospital 26, 27
child assessment orders 235–6
childhood diseases 1–3, 10
  reasons for admission to hospital 34–7
children
  activities in hospital 38–41
    play, *see* play
  admitted to adult wards 25, 33–4, 76
  chronic sickness, *see* chronically sick children
  compliance with treatment, *see* cooperation
  consent 43, 225–6, 227–8
    by proxy 228–9
    exploring implications 228–9
    Gillick competence 233–4
    participation in research 227
  health expenditure on 30
  length of stay in hospital 32
    aiding normal development 66
    behaviour problems 86
  levels of understanding 43
    afterlife 129–31, 134
    body parts and functions 44–5
    death 126–9
    health 45
    illness 46–9
    intent of treatment 48, 49

justice and punishment 2, 47–8, 49, 107, 108, 189
life-threatening conditions 131–4
pain 106–8
surgical procedures 177
mortality rates 1, 4, 6
numbers of hospital admissions 30–2, 33
parental attachment to 4
preparation for hospitalization 73–4
  age of child 79, 80
  booklets 78
  explanation 81
  gender of child 79
  home visits 75
  modelling 77–8
  painful and unpleasant procedures 77
  photographs 78
  planned admissions 74–5
  play 78
  previous medical experience 79–80
  questions 80–1
  talking 79
  timing 80
  unfamiliar sensations 77
  unplanned admissions 75–6
reasons for admission to hospital 34–7, 38
refusal of treatment 234–5
reluctance to treat 2, 4
removal from parental custody 321
rights in institutions 238–42
separation from parents 13–14, 16–19; *see also* visiting restrictions
  Bowlby's attachment theory 19–20
  discontinuity 86–7
  effects in later childhood 22–4
welfare rights 26–7, 233
Children Act 1989 43, 228, 231, 232–4
  protection orders 235–7
children's hospitals
  age restrictions 8, 9
  continental Europe 1, 7
  history 1, 5–9
    daily life 11
    diet 10
    payment for treatment 9–10
    results 12–13
    staffing 11–12
    treatment 11
  United States 9, 11
  views for and against 6–7, 13
  visiting, *see* visiting restrictions
Chimney Sweeps Act 1840 5